Trauma in Dentistry

Edited by Serdar Gözler

Published in London, United Kingdom

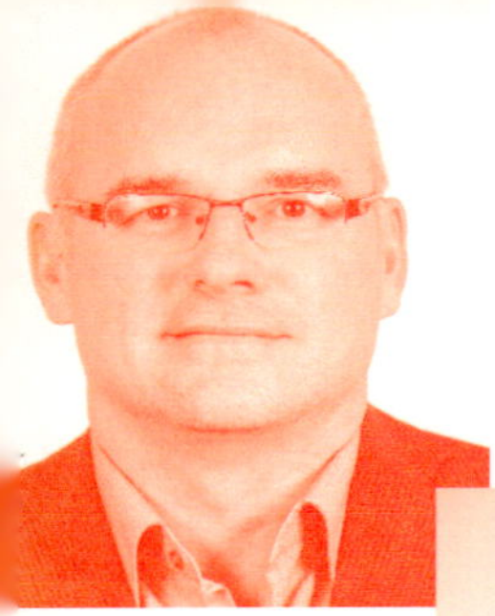
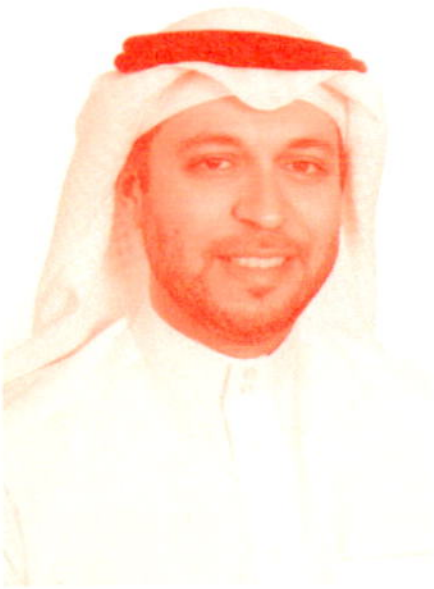
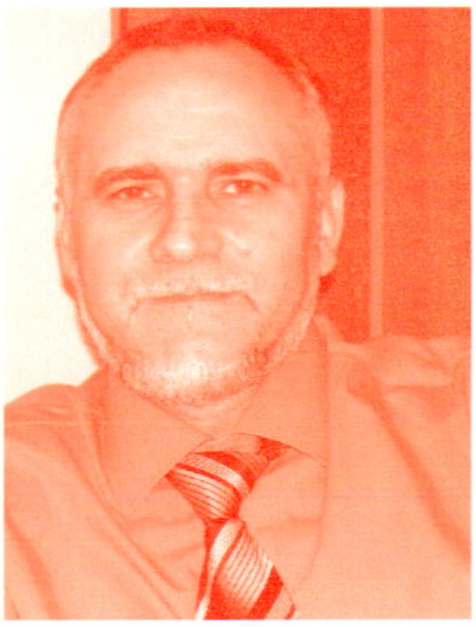
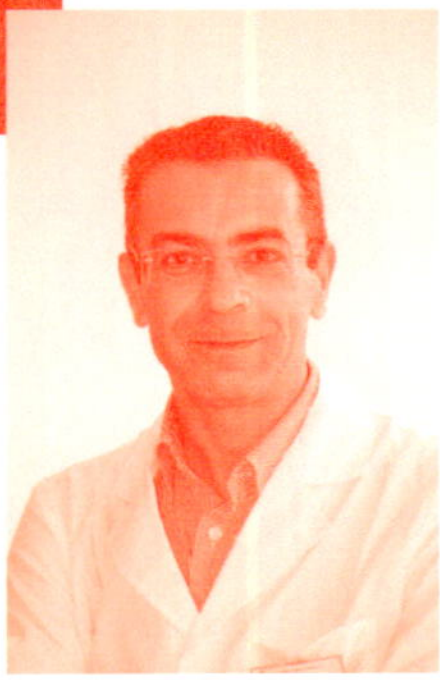
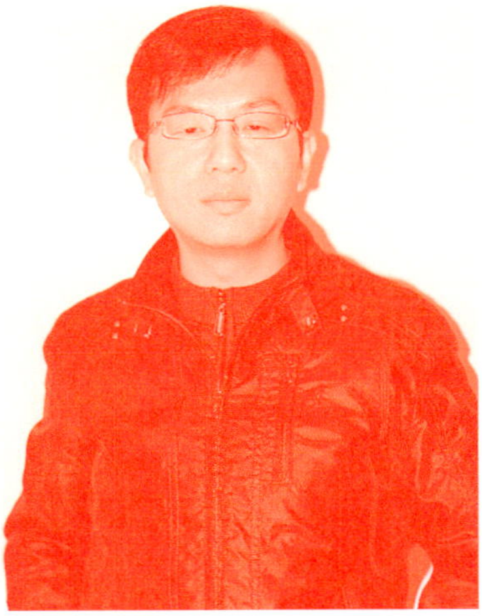
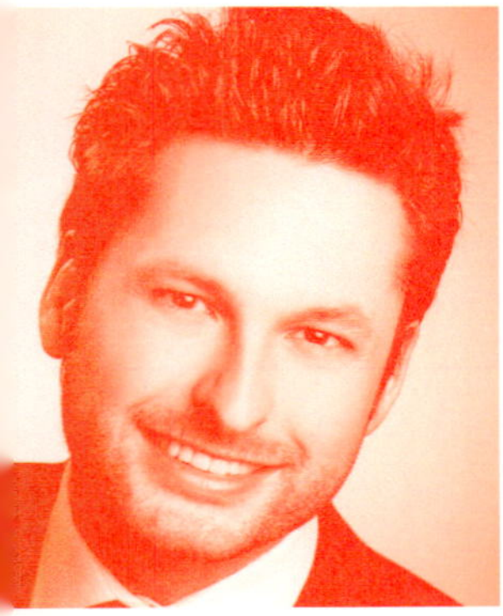
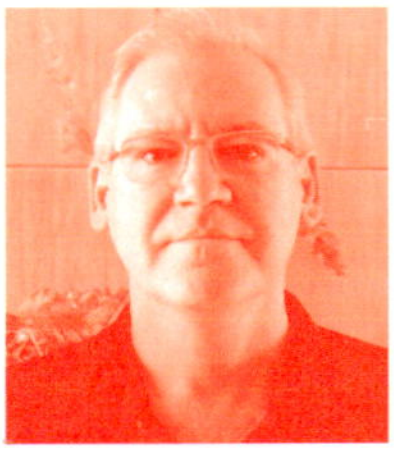

IntechOpen

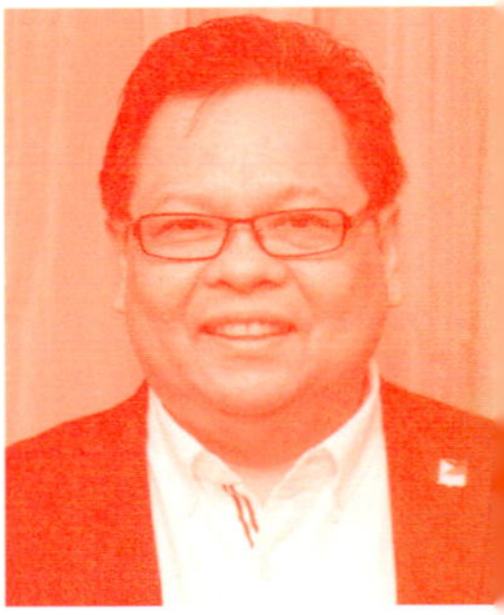
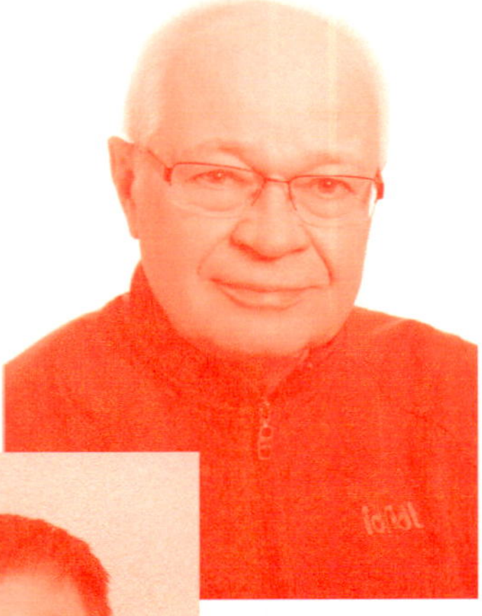
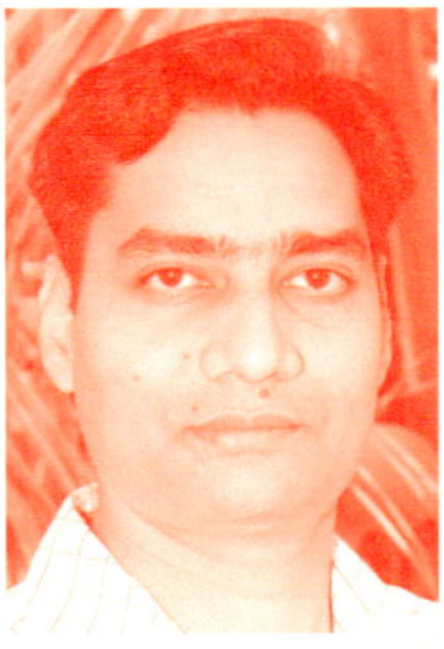
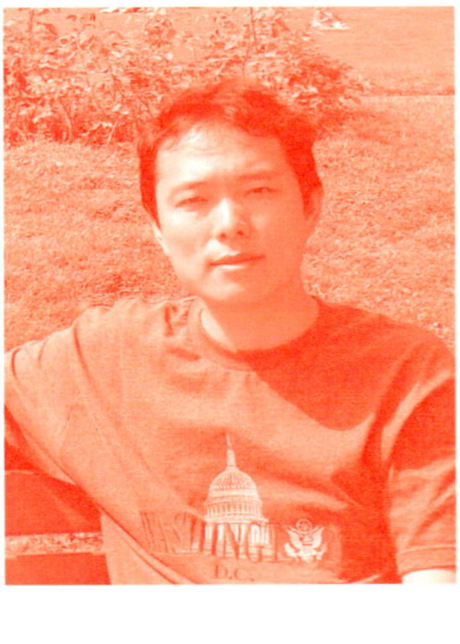
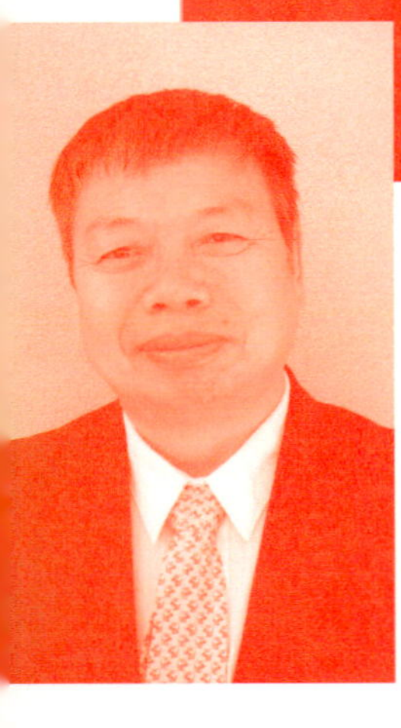
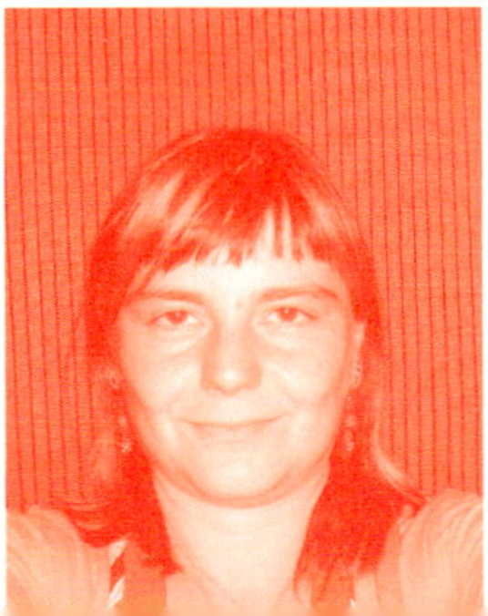

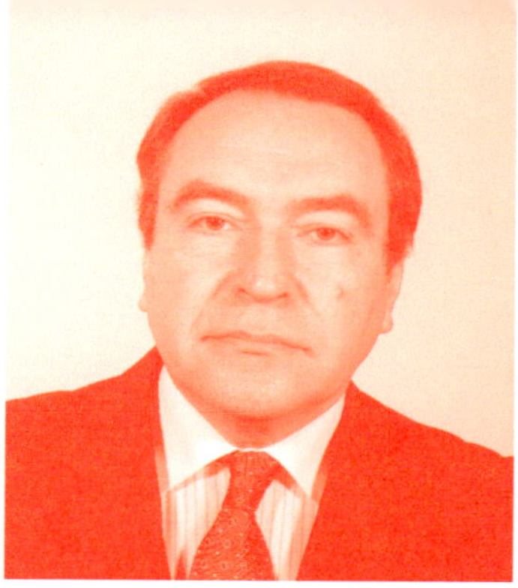
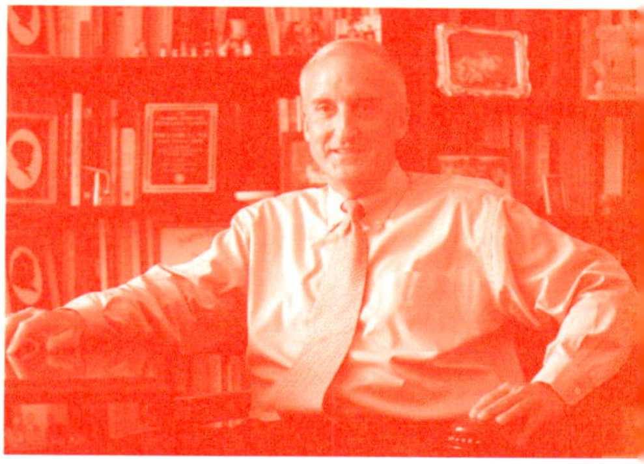
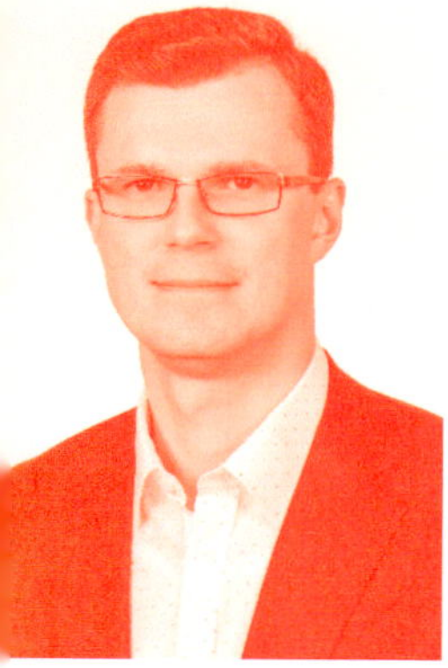
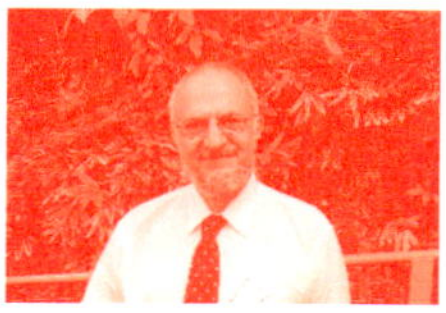
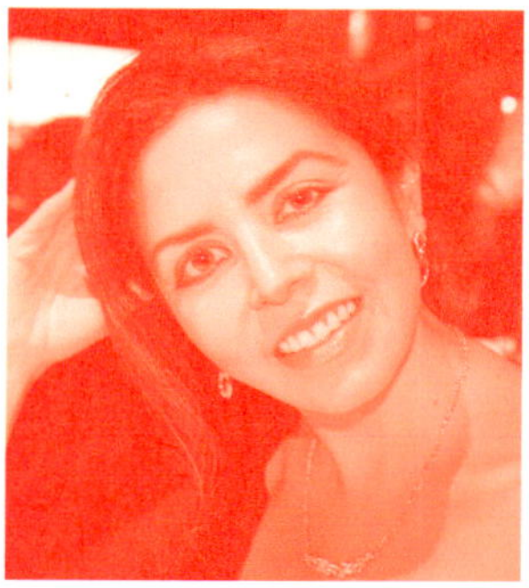

Supporting open minds since 2005

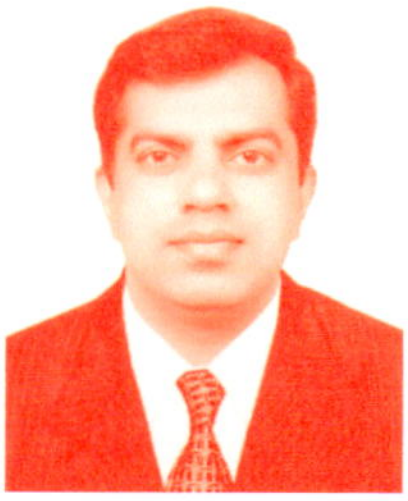
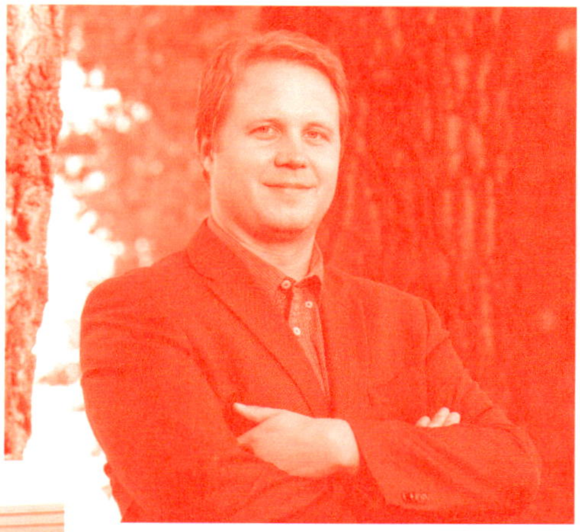
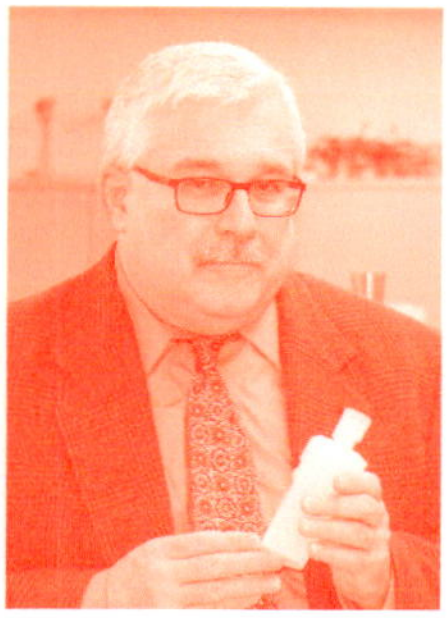
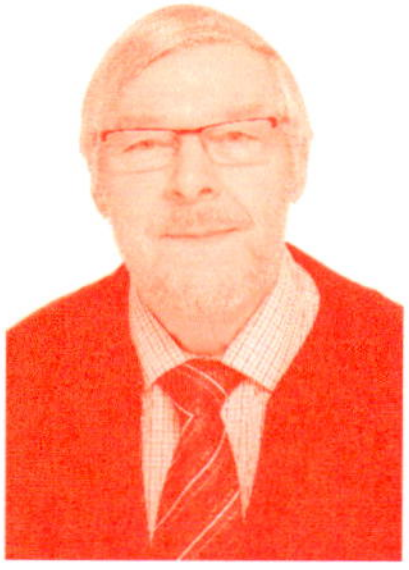
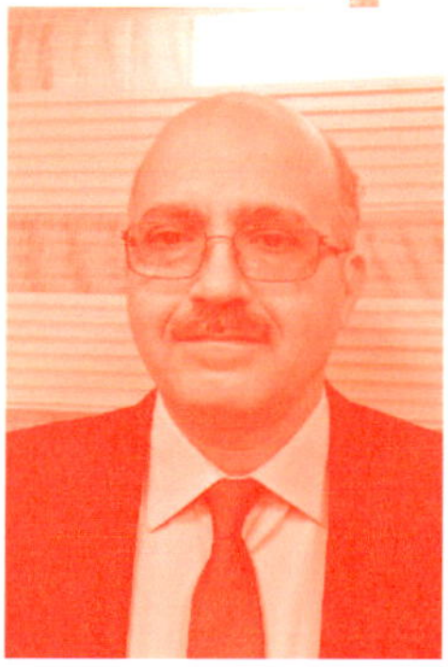
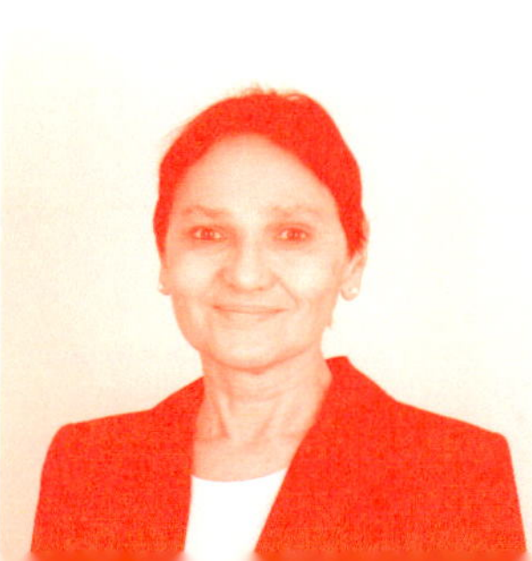
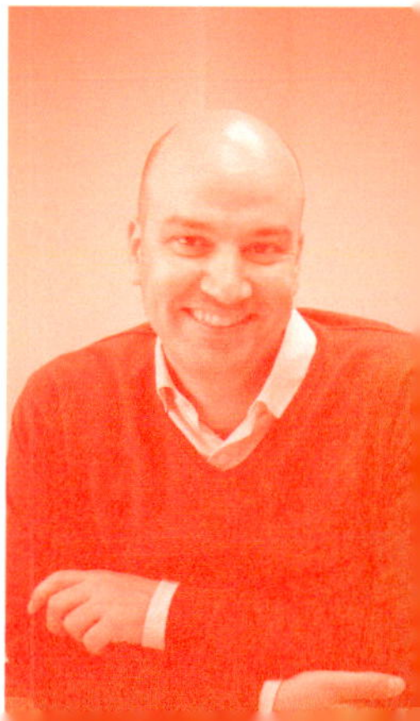

Trauma in Dentistry
http://dx.doi.org/10.5772/intechopen.77126
Edited by Serdar Gözler

Part of IntechOpen Book Series: Dentistry, Volume 3
Book Series Editor: Zühre Akarslan

Contributors
Sanaz Sadry, Tosun Tosun, Meltem Koray, Aslı Topaloglu-Ak, Pinar Karataban, Didem Oner Ozdas, Sevgi Zorlu, Mehmet Yaltirik, Humeyra Kocaelli, Duygu Ofluoglu, Cevat Tugrul Turgut, Guhan Dergin, Yusuf Emes, Buket Aybar, Serdar Gözler

First published in London, United Kingdom, 2019 by IntechOpen
IntechOpen is the global imprint of INTECHOPEN LIMITED, registered in England and Wales, registration number: 11086078, The Shard, 25th floor, 32 London Bridge Street
London, SE19SG - United Kingdom
Printed in Croatia

British Library Cataloguing-in-Publication Data
A catalogue record for this book is available from the British Library

Additional hard and PDF copies can be obtained from orders@intechopen.com

Trauma in Dentistry
Edited by Serdar Gözler
p. cm.
Print ISBN 978-1-78985-626-2
Online ISBN 978-1-83881-127-3
eBook (PDF) ISBN 978-1-83881-128-0

For EU product safety concerns:
IN TECH d.o.o., Prolaz Marije Krucifikse Kozulić 3, 51000 Rijeka, Croatia, info@intechopen.com or visit our website at intechopen.com.

IntechOpen Book Series

Dentistry

Volume 3

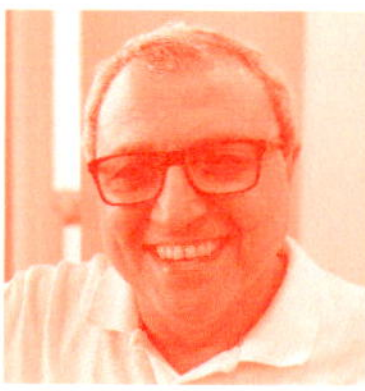

Dr. Serdar Gözler was born in Adana, Turkey, in 1956. He completed his undergraduate studies at the Faculty of Dentistry at Marmara University, Istanbul, Turkey in 1978. and obtained his PhD from the Istanbul and Dicle University in Turkey in 1982. He has published papers in international and national scientific journals, book chapters, and research articles on occlusion and temporomandibular joint disorders. Dr. Gözler is currently Director of the Temporomandibular Joint Disorders Department at Istanbul Aydın University.

Editor of Volume 3: Serdar Gözler
Istanbul Aydin University, Turkey

Book Series Editor: Zühre Akarslan
Gazi University Faculty of Dentistry, Turkey

Scope of the Series

The major pathologies which dentists encounter in clinical practice include dental caries and periodontal diseases. Diagnosis and treatment of these pathologies is essential because when untreated, abscess could occur and it can even lead to the extraction of the tooth. Extracted teeth can be replaced with implants. Dentists and patients are nowadays more familiar with dental implant treatments. As a result, advanced diagnostic tools which aid in pre-operative treatment planning (cone-beam computed tomography, computer aided implant planning etc..), new implant designs improving the success of osteointegration, new materials, and techniques are introduced in the dental market.
Conditions which dentists frequently encounter in their clinical practice are temporomandibular joint (TMJ) disorders. These disorders include degenerative musculoskeletal conditions associated with morphological and functional deformities. Accurate diagnosis is important for proper management of TMJ pathologies. With the advance in technology, new materials, techniques and equipment are introduced in the dental practice. New diagnostic aids in dental caries detection, cone-beam computed tomographic imaging, soft and hard tissue lasers, advances in oral and maxillofacial surgery procedures, uses of ultrasound, CAD/CAM, nanotechnology, plasma rich protein (PRP) and dental implantology are some of them. There will be even more new applications in dentistry in the future.
This book series includes topics related to dental caries, dentomaxillofacial imaging, new trends in oral implantology, new approaches in oral and maxillofacial surgery, temporomandibular joint disorders in dentistry etc.

Contents

Preface

Trauma in Dentistry is written by academics who specialize in the field, but in no way do we claim that this book covers all issues related to the subject.

Many of the academic issues that are thought to be theoretical in essence are, in fact, thoroughly in the clinical environment. Even though the practices of surgical, prosthetic, and restorative dentistry fundamentally cover conventional procedures, post-traumatic treatment differs from classical approaches in the sense that it requires more advanced diagnostic and treatment techniques. Many of the post-trauma-related treatments especially are as combined surgical and restorative treatments in contemporary dentistry. This is the type of experience that the academics who have contributed to this volume have. This volume not only covers the scientific basis of trauma and trauma-related matters, but it also aims to draw attention to these advanced diagnostic and treatment methods that may be used for dealing with dental trauma.

The most important matter regarding post-trauma treatment is to diagnose quickly and correctly and implement the right treatment. This volume includes information regarding both adult and pediatric treatments, as children make up the largest portion of the dental trauma population. We hope this volume will pioneer much-advanced publications in the field of traumatic dental injuries.

Another important issue to consider besides traumatic injuries is occlusal traumas. Therefore we dedicate a chapter to this topic that covers neuromuscular foundations and the most up-to-date treatment methods available.

Aside from the information on diagnostic and treatment techniques, this volume includes information on biomaterials. I especially hope the content on the features of biological restorative materials and their application techniques will be helpful for clinical practice.

Also covered in this book is one of the more routine practices of dentistry, that is, implant treatments. Though there are numerous publications on the matter, this book not only draws attention to the relationship between implants and traumatic cases that dentists frequently come across, but it also discusses potential treatment methods available.

I believe that all my colleagues, who have not only encouraged me but who have also taken the time and effort to prepare this volume, have given their utmost with complete sincerity.

I would also like to thank my wife who has shown appreciation and understanding for all the time I devoted to preparing this book for publication.

Serdar Gözler
Istanbul Aydin University,
Turkey

Section 1

Introduction

Chapter 1

Introductory Chapter: Etiology, Diagnostic, and Treatment Procedure at Traumatic Cases in Dentistry

Serdar Gözler

1. Introduction

Dental trauma presents one of the most important situations where clinicians are called upon to make unscheduled diagnostic and treatment approaches in an area that is outside their routine experience. Guidelines have been outlined for management of numerous dental and medical conditions. Traumatic cases in dentistry are classified by many sources; however, the World Health Organization's (WHO) classification system is the most comprehensive system which allows for minimal subjective interpretations. The WHO traumatic classification system is built up according to the following situations [1]:

1. Fracture of enamel of tooth,
2. Fracture of crown without pulpal involvement,
3. Fracture of crown with pulpal involvement,
4. Fracture of root of tooth,
5. Fracture of crown together with the root,
6. Unspecified tooth fracture,
7. Tooth luxation,
8. Intrusion and/or extrusion of teeth
9. Avulsion of teeth,
10. Other type of injuries including burns and laceration.

Most of the reported traumatic cases come from falls while children play [2]. At the present time, the dental trauma term must also be included for dental treatment sourced from traumatic cases. There are various invasive restorative dental treatment models in modern dentistry at the present time. For example, dental implant treatments, tissue repair purpose treatments, augmentations of maxillary sinuses, and full mouth ceramic restoration treatments are restorative treatments which have extreme trauma risks.

Traumatic cases need urgent diagnosis and quick treatment. However, according to a review article by Andrease et al., there are few studies showing a positive relationship between treatment delay and pulpal and periodontal ligament healing complications [3]. Practical and most economic reasons are fulfilled such as demand for acute treatment (i.e. within a few hours) or delayed (i.e. after the first 24 hours) in traumatic cases. But it is commonly accepted that all injuries should be treated within few hours, for the comfort of the patient and also to reduce wound healing complications.

Another type of dental trauma is post-op developed traumatic cases which are based on bad occlusion usually. In many cases, sinus augmentation may be necessary; in this case, augmented sinus tissue must be supported by a biomaterial. Implants are placed when the biomaterial is set like a wall. The implants will bear occlusal forces after finishing implant-supported crowns. In some cases, biomaterial wall cannot bear the occlusal forces of implant-supported crowns and then collapses. That kind of problems is related to premature contact originated occlusal trauma. Traumatic occlusion is the most important reason for the breaking of the restorations or collapse of the operating area under the pressure of high occlusal load. Early occlusal contacts force the area with all cumulative occlusal pressure of the jaws. There may not be a problem if there is an adequate thickness set at the sinus augmentation. But in some cases, under the high occlusal forces, the biomaterial wall cannot bear the load and collapses consequently. Sometimes, sinus wall tears and the implant is mobilized to the far side of the sinus. The first action must take out the dislocated implant from the exposed sinus and repair the sinus wall. Generally, the accepted protocol is to wait after repair of the sinus area and then continue the implant treatment again [4, 5]. There are various approaches for the planning of dental implants: the number of implants, their locations, inclinations, quality of supporting bone, etc. In its wider sense, this includes considerations of multiple inter-related factors of ensuring adequate bone support, implant location number, length, distribution, and inclination, splinting, vertical dimension esthetics, occlusal schemes, and more [6]. Every different alternative of the planning of implant treatment will have a different effect on implant-supported restoration. The difference is related to the occlusal scheme of the prosthetic restoration.

Dentists must take their decisions according to their past experiences because the patients in avulsion are rare except children patients and emergency patients [7]. Additionally, clinicians must trust the preparation guidelines for trauma standards and the protocols stated before.

The protocols are set before but they have not tested for prospectively longitudinal studies in human. However, all protocols are set before and have found a strong place for routine applications clinically.

Periodontal wound healing protocols must be taken specially and must be based on biological reasons.

Permanent teeth's avulsions are the most serious of all dental traumatic cases. The prognosis of the treatment depends on the time taken at the place of accident or the time immediately after the avulsion [7]. Appropriate emergency management and treatment plan are important for a good prognosis. Guidelines are usually useful for delivering the best treatment possible in an efficient manner. The International Association of Dental Traumatology (IADT) has developed a consensus statement after a review of the dental literature and group discussions.

Unlike deciduous teeth, permanent teeth rarely undergo root resorption. Even in the presence of periodontal and radicular inflammation, resorption will occur primarily on the support bone side of the attachment apparatus and the root will be resistant to it [8].

Facial trauma that results in fractured, displaced, or lost teeth (deciduous or permanent) can have significant negative functional, esthetic, and psychological effects on children. Clinicians should collaborate to educate the children and parents about the prevention and treatment of traumatic injuries to the oral and maxillofacial area.

2. Diagnosis and treatment procedures according to the types of the traumatic cases

2.1 Radiographic examination

Several radiographic images must be taken from every patient in different angles, but the final decision is up to the clinician [9].

The following are suggested:

- X-ray image with 90° parallel with central rays through the examined tooth.
- Occlusal radiological examination.
- A lateral angulated dental periapical image which includes the mesial or distal aspects of the teeth examined as much as possible.

Cone-beam computerized tomography is extremely useful at this stage. It can be used for radiographic examination in detail of root fractures, mobility of teeth, periodontal status, and peripheral destructions of teeth. The CBT Radiographic System may not be available in every clinic; it may not be used routinely, but advantages of the system cannot be compared with those of conventional systems. Information for dental application of CBT is documented very well in the scientific literature.

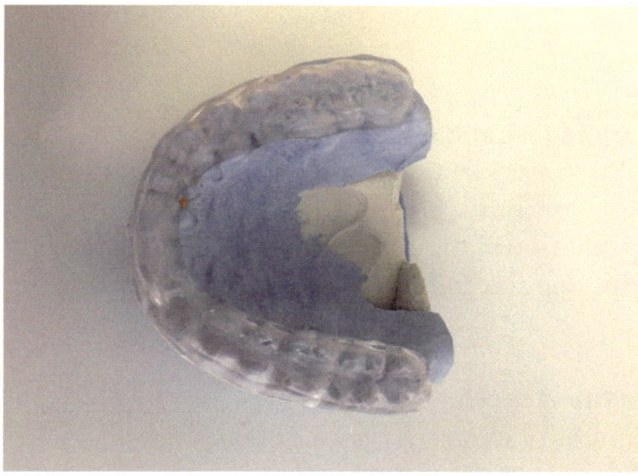

Figure 1.
Nonrigid splints can be used for stabilization of mobilized and fractured teeth.

2.2 Clinical examination, basic principles, and suggestions

There are many protocols and approaches to the clinical examination. They are very well classified and documented in current textbooks for assessment of TDIs [1].

2.3 Fixation with splints and their using period

According to the recent researches, using short-term nonrigid splints for treatment of luxated, fractured, and avulsed teeth is supported (**Figure 1**). Basically, splints are essentials for the patient's comfort and improvement of functions, and they are useful to maintain the location and correct position of teeth [9–11].

2.4 Medical treatment, antibiotics

There is no strong evidence for using systemic antibiotics for traumatic cases, luxation management, and coverage improvement of root fractures of teeth. This option is not mandatory and it is up to the dentist's own decision according to the past experience. Root fractures and related injures of teeth and soft tissue may need surgical intervention. Use of antibiotic option is harmonized to the surgical operations and especially it may be useful for the soft tissue healing procedure [12, 7]. Soft tissue injuries, treatment methods, and healing procedure information are neither comprehensive nor detailed information is found in textbooks, the scientific literature, and, most recently, the Dental Trauma Guide (DTG) that can be accessed on http://www.dentaltraumaguide.org. Additionally, the DTG, also available on the IADT's web page http://www.iadt-dentaltrauma.org, provides a visual and animated documentation of treatment procedures as well as estimations of prognosis for the various TDIs [13].

2.5 Use of antibiotics

There is no strong evidence for using systemic antibiotics for traumatic cases, luxation management, and coverage improvement of root fractures of teeth. This option is not mandatory and it is up to the dentist's own decision according to the past experience. Root fractures and related injures of teeth and soft tissue may need surgical intervention. Use of antibiotic option is harmonized to the surgical operations and especially it may be useful for soft the tissue healing procedure [14, 15, 2, 16].

2.6 Sensitivity tests

Sensitivity tests (cold test and electrical pulp test) are necessary for improving the pulp condition. Especially in an emergency atmosphere of a traumatic condition, revealing of pulp condition is one of the important attempts for treatment steps. Therefore, at least two signs and symptoms are necessary to make the diagnosis of necrotic pulp. Regular follow-up controls are required to make a pulpal diagnosis.

2.7 Vitality of permanent teeth

The basic principle is that maximum endeavor should be made for the protection of pulp vitality in a permanent tooth improving root development. Loss of a tooth in the period of childhood will produce occlusal source many complications. The immature permanent tooth can recover easily after exposing the pulp in traumatic tooth/root fractures. In traumatic cases, root canal treatments are the most reasonable treatment for maintaining root development [8]. Additionally, emergency treatment of traumatized teeth can accelerate healing of the teeth.

2.8 Traumatic occlusion

As a dental practitioner, we may cause occlusal trauma. We change the occlusal surfaces of teeth when we make functional and esthetical restorations in clinical practice. Usually, natural teeth have adapted and shaped occlusion in the developmental period of humans, especially the development of the craniofacial area [17]. Muscles, bones, and teeth must be in full harmony. But sometimes, they may not be in accordance with accepted rules or standards, especially anatomically. The neural system also adapts to that inappropriate structure and there does not exist any high neuronal impulse in the neural system that may cause excessive contraction of masticatory muscles [18]. The dentist may change this complex, improper but harmonic structure. Dental treatment procedures may disrupt this harmonic relationship when we make composite restoration, orthodontic treatment, prosthetic, and/or implant restoration. In order to avoid traumatic occlusion, occlusal compliance in dental restorations should be at the highest possible level.

Occlusal trauma may be spotted in the following situations:

1. Prosthetic restorations

2. Implant supported prosthesis

3. Composite fillings

4. Orthodontic treatment

5. Oral surgery operations

6. Accidents

The main reason for the occlusal trauma is premature contact in the occlusion. Every dentist must be able to manage premature contacts in dental treatments.

Occlusal trauma is one of the most common problems of dental treatment. Every dentist must be extremely careful about avoiding dental premature contacts.

Trauma itself is not a disturbance, trauma is a result of an event. *Trauma is the damage of tissue and/or organs.* Trauma and its consequences may be acute or chronic. The acute situation is the result of the quick reflex response of the neuromuscular system to the premature contacts; however, the chronic situation may be developed within days, weeks, or years. The perception of the occlusal irregularity and a reaction to that problem is managed by the central nervous system (CNS). During human life, the main function of the masticatory muscles is to break food down into pieces small enough to be swallowed. CNS is like a protection mechanism of the stomatognathic system in that function. These are strong muscles that generate very large forces across in very short distances and apply them via rigid teeth. Such large forces can easily damage the teeth and their supporting tissues, tongue, cheeks, and the joints unless they are controlled precisely and effectively [3]. If the trauma is a system for protection of the stomatognathic structures, pain is the alarm ring bell of that system.

One of the biggest problems of prosthetic restorations is occlusal premature contacts. Early occlusal contacts cause the imbalance of dentures and it may fracture the ceramic restorations. Unbalanced dentures are the reason for occlusal trauma and they may cause irritation on soft tissue and then tissue deteriorations consequently (**Figure 2**).

Occlusal premature contacts are effective on the way from the first contact to the maximum intercuspal position (MIP). It is not easy to detect premature contact at developing occlusion (**Figure 3**).

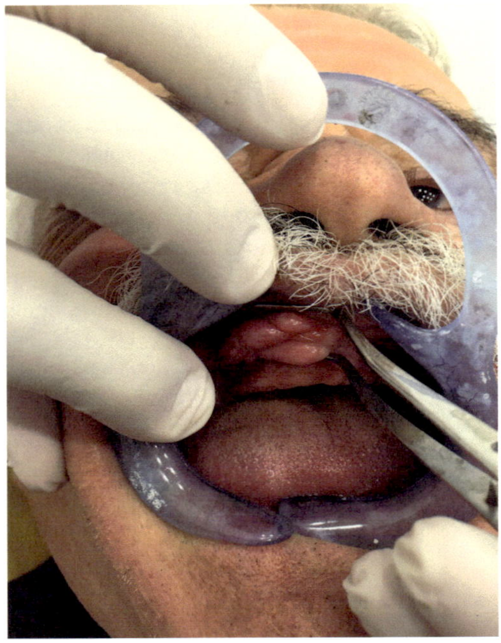

Figure 2.
Occlusal trauma caused by an upper denture.

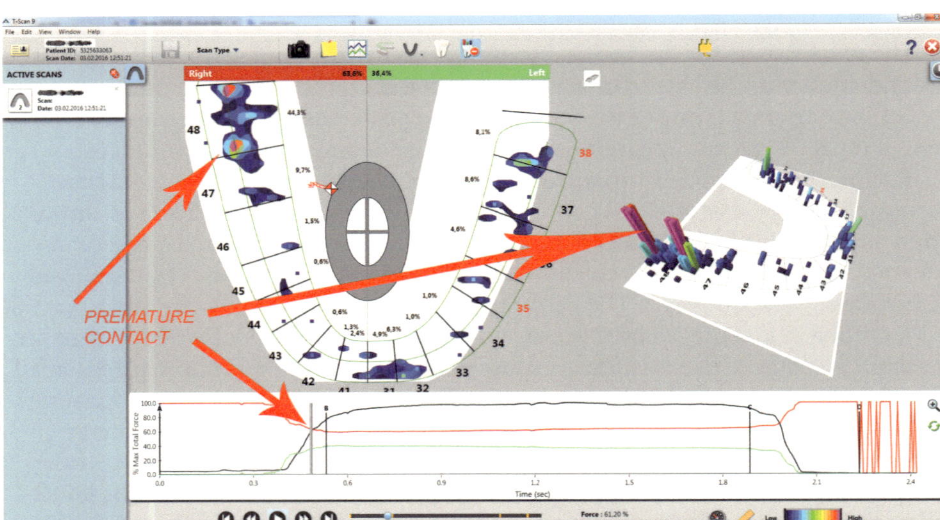

Figure 3.
Occlusal trauma: premature contact is affected on the way before of the way of MIP (maximum intercuspal position) peak point.

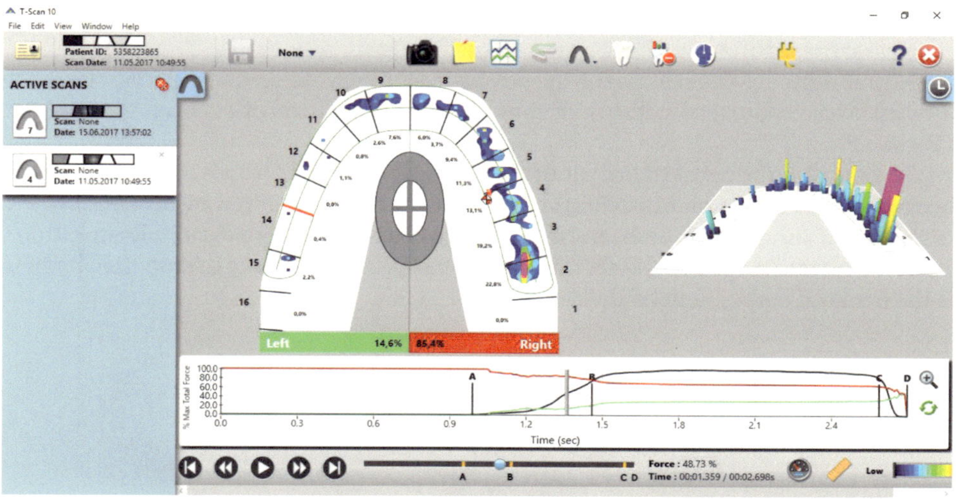

Figure 4.
Premature contacts can be described easily by computerized occlusal analyzing system. Occlusal papers or similar methods can not much help for finding premature contact.

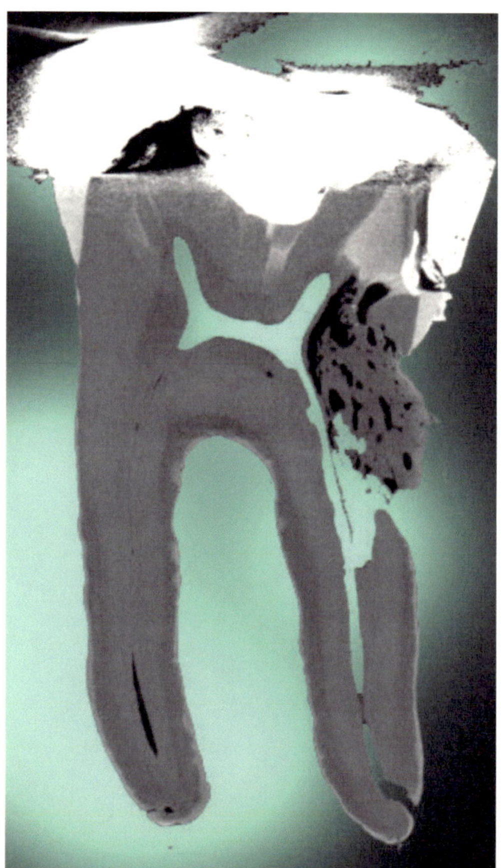

Figure 5.
Cervical area of a tooth has been destroyed under the traumatic occlusion.

The best method is computerized occlusal analyzing system for detecting the traumatic premature contact (**Figure 4**).

Abfractions are the reason for the wrong linear inclination of teeth and the tooth cervical area is damaged because of those kinds of problems of occlusal trauma (**Figure 5**).

Sometimes, the cervical area at the labial surface of the tooth is abraded in time because of the direction of occlusal force. If the teeth are covered by ceramic crown restoration, abrasion of teeth continues inside the ceramic restoration. Restorations are not protective against the abrasion (**Figure 6**). The only way to stop the abrasion is the occlusal adjustment of the restoration.

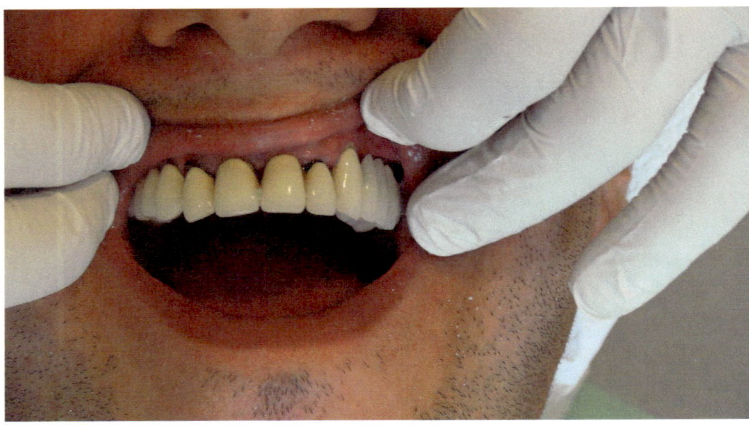

Figure 6.
Abfraction continues under the restorations. Crown restorations cannot protect the teeth from traumatic occlusal forces.

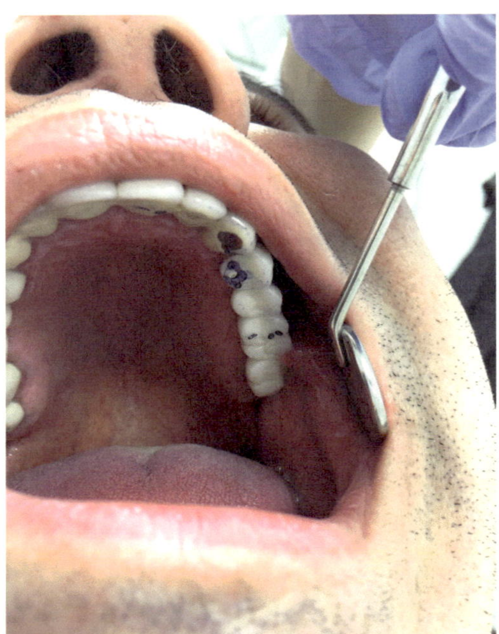

Figure 7.
Ceramic restorations have been broken under the traumatic occlusal strokes.

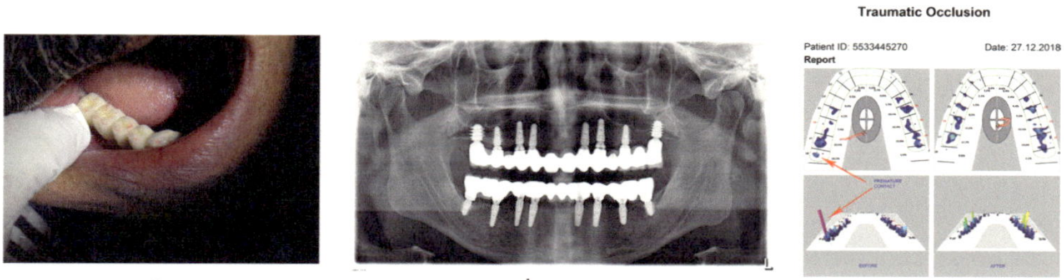

a b c

Figure 8.
(a–c) Implant selection, their locations, and surgical steps are almost perfect; (a) everything seems normal when controlling with articulating paper, (b) but the patient is never relaxed with his new restorations. The problem can be detected when examining restoration with computerized occlusal analysis technic: there is severe premature contact detected on the right second molar area (c). The patient relaxed just after occlusal adjustment (c).

The ceramic materials are often used in restorative treatments. Premature contacts on the ceramic restorations must be eliminated; otherwise, periodontal receptors will never stop sending neuronal impulse and the muscles will never be relaxed. In this case, ceramic restoration has been broken because of the high occlusal pressure of premature contacts (**Figure** 7).

The abrasion effect of occlusal trauma is much more dramatically developed in the cases of implant prosthesis because implant restorations have no resilient features and the force transmits directly to the bone without resistance of any force breaker system like periodontal ligaments of natural teeth. In an implant-supported prosthesis, if occlusal equilibration is not made, the patient can never be relaxed. In **Figure 8a** and **b**, implant planning and surgery phase is perfect and the treatment with a full arch ceramic restoration is also finished, but the patient is never relaxed with his new restorations. The problem can be detected when examining restoration with computerized occlusal analysis technic: there is severe premature contact detected on the right second molar area. The patient relaxed just after an occlusal adjustment procedure (**Figure 8c**).

3. Conclusion

The most exposed group to dental trauma is young adults and children. Fractures of the upper part of the teeth and luxations are the most frequent cases. For a healthy result, the most important approach is the proper diagnosis and then proper treatment consequently.. This action plan is not only for tooth level, but is also a proper approach for other type traumatic injuries; the guidelines which have been developed and set by "The International Association of Dental Traumatology (IADT)" are important supportive materials for the clinicians. There are many specialists and researchers on "Dental Traumatology" who added important and useful suggestions.

In some cases, the collected data from traumatic injury may not be clear and precise. In those cases, clinicians can use the basic and agreed of opinions of IADT board specialists. Suggestions and opinions for unexpected situations are also developed by the IDTA members.

There are various guidelines for any kind of levels of urgent and long-term traumatic cases which are prepared and set by TDIs.

Author details

Serdar Gözler
Prosthodontic Department of Dentistry Faculty, Istanbul Aydın University, Istanbul, Turkey

*Address all correspondence to: serdargozler@aydin.edu.tr

References

[1] Bastone EB, Freer TJ, Mcnamara JR. Epidemiology of dental trauma: A review of the literature. Australian Dental Journal. 2000;**45**(1)

[2] Perez R, Berkowitz R, Mcllveen L, Forrester D. Dental trauma in children: A survey. Dental Traumatology. 1991;**7**(5):212-213. DOI: 10.1111/j.1600-9657.1991.tb00438.x

[3] Andreasen JO, Gerds TA, Lauridsen E, Ahrensburg SS. Dental trauma guide a source of evidence-based treatment guidelines for dental trauma. Dental Traumatology. 2012;**28**:345-350

[4] Cotruţă AM, Mihăescu CS, Tănăsescu LA, Mărgărit R, Andrei OC. Analyzing the morphology and intensity of occlusal contacts in implant-prosthetic restorations using t-scan system. Romanian Journal of Morphology and Embryology. 2015;**56**(1):277-281

[5] Wong RCW, Tideman H, Kin L, Merkx MAW. Biomechanics of mandibular reconstruction: A review. International Journal of Oral and Maxillofacial Surgery. 2010;**39**(4):313-319. DOI: 10.1016/j.ijom.2009.11.003

[6] Gross MD. Occlusion in implant dentistry. A review of the literature of prosthetic determinants and current concepts. Australian Dental Journal. 2008;**53**(Suppl. 1)

[7] Flores MT, Andersson L, Andreasen JO, Bakland LK, Malmgren B, Barnett F, et al. Guidelines for the management of traumatic dental injuries. II. Avulsion of permanent teeth. Dental Traumatology. 2007;**23**(3):130-136

[8] Trope M. Root resorption due to dental trauma. Endodontic Topics. 2002

[9] Diangelis AJ, Andreasen JO, Ebeleseder KA, Kenny DJ, Trope M, Sigurdsson A, et al. Guidelines for the management of traumatic dental injuries: 1. Fractures and luxations of permanent teeth. Pediatric Dentistry. 2016;**38**(6):358-368

[10] Flores MT, Malmgren B, Andersson L, Andreasen JO, Bakland LK, Barnett F, et al. Guidelines for the management of traumatic dental injuries. III. Primary teeth. Dental Traumatology. 2007;**23**(4):196-202

[11] Von Arx T, Filippi A, Lussi A. Comparison of a new dental trauma splint device (TTS) with three commonly used splinting techniques. Dental Traumatology. 2001;**17**(6):266-274

[12] Lin S, Zuckerman O, Fuss Z, Ashkenazi M. New emphasis in the treatment of dental trauma: Avulsion and luxation. Dental Traumatology. 2007;**23**(5):297-303

[13] Berger TD, Kenny DJ, Casas MJ, Barrett EJ, Lawrence HP. Effects of severe dentoalveolar trauma on the quality-of-life of children and parents. Dental Traumatology. 2009;**25**(5):462-469. DOI: 10.1111/j.1600-9657.2009.00809.x

[14] Lee JY, Yanpiset K, Sigurdsson A, Vann WF. A case report of reattachment of fractured root fragment and resin-composite reinforcement in a compromised endodontically treated root. Dental Traumatology. 2001;**17**(5):227-230

[15] Kargul B, Caglar E, Tanboga I. Dental trauma in Turkish children, Istanbul. Dental Traumatology. 2003;**19**(2):72-75. DOI: 10.1034/j.1600-9657.2003.00091.x

[16] Case I, De Rossi SS, Stern I, Sollecito TP, Fushima K, Gallo LM, et al. Dislocation of the. Journal of Prosthodontic Research.

1985;**25**(3):246-251. DOI: 10.1016/j.jfoodeng.2016.06.008

[17] Hattori Y, Satoh C, Kunieda T, Endoh R, Hisamatsu H, Watanabe M. Bite forces and their resultants during forceful intercuspal clenching in humans. Journal of Biomechanics. 2009;**42**(10):1533-1538

[18] Iwase M, Ohashi M, Tachibana H, Toyoshima T, Nagumo M. Bite force, occlusal contact area and masticatory efficiency before and after orthognathic surgical correction of mandibular prognathism. International Journal of Oral and Maxillofacial Surgery. 2006;**35**(12):1102-1107

Section 2

Implants

Chapter 2

Dental Implants and Trauma

Tosun Tosun and Koray Meltem

Abstract

Implant dentistry treatment target to avoid any kind of edentulous state including tooth loss due to trauma. In the literature there are numerous case reports and few clinical studies documenting treatment options of post-trauma patients by dental implants. Principally there are some limitations of dental implant application related to the age and available bone volume of patients. Implant candidate should complete bone growth as the metallic implants do not follow bony development phases. Most often traumatic dental injuries occur in childhood and implant treatment should postponed. In this aspect the major problem associated with dental implant placement is the lack of adequate bone volumes at the future time of surgery as such cases receives traumatic dental injury in the early years and disuse atrophy occurs during waiting period. Future trends and strategies in dental traumatology in general and with special attention to dental implant applications are based on the education of population in terms of emergency treatments and urgent transport of patients to the clinics.

Keywords: dental implant, trauma, implant placement, dental lasers, erbium laser, traumatic injuries, iatrogenic factors

1. Introduction

Dental implant applications are wide spreading globally and in last three decades it is the major attraction field for both clinicians and patients. Implant dentistry treatments target to avoid any kind of edentulous state including tooth loss due to trauma. Tooth loss after trauma could be related to traumatic dental injuries depending from violence, falls, traffic accidents, gunshots or to late consequences of trauma such as recurrent endodontic lesions, vertical root fractures, external or internal root resorptions and ankylosis which bring teeth to untreatable condition. Trauma-related tooth loss most often involve anterior maxillary teeth and generally is rehabilitated as single tooth implant replacement or several teeth are affected and rehabilitation is made as a solution of partially edentulous case but being in the anterior region with the rules of single-tooth replacement to preserve esthetics. Patient age constitute another aspect of post-trauma cases where accidents mainly happen in childhood period which is not favorable for dental implant applications due to incomplete bony growth. For the patients in development stage there should be followed special attention for future dental implant rehabilitation. Thus, care must be taken to find suitable treatment solutions in order to provide interim prosthetic treatment, to follow normal bone growth, avoid hard tissue atrophy and preserve alveolar bony dimensions for upcoming implant surgery in the late adolescent age. In the present chapter post-trauma applications of dental implants are discussed and possible treatment strategies are evaluated.

2. Etiology, prevalence of traumatic dental injuries and implant dentistry

Traumatic dental injuries (TDIs) have different frequencies worldwide, but always low prevalence among communities [1–6]. Etiologic factors of TDIs are various from country to country and with age groups [7]. Globally the most common etiology of TDI in men is violence. For women there are three most common injury factors: violence, falls and traffic injuries [6, 8–10]. Ballistic injuries (gunshots) form a severe type of traumatic maxillofacial injury [11, 12] and can be classified in between the etiologic factors of TDIs. TDI studies most often cover children and adolescents. There are few studies involving adults [1, 6, 13, 14]. Studies show that the TDIs affect mainly anterior maxilla and especially central incisors [3, 8, 15–17]. Generally teeth involved by TDIs are lost in the long run and subsequently this anatomic lack may result in significant esthetic and functional problems [6].

The consensus statements of International Association of Dental Traumatology (IADT) propose to delineate approaches for the immediate or urgent care for management of primary and permanent teeth injuries [9, 10, 18]. The emergency treatment after TDIs is highly important for the future management of dental structures [15, 16]. Although attempts is to preserve natural dentition and despite best efforts at retaining and maintaining trauma-compromised teeth, studies show that in the long run affected teeth are loose and replaced by dental implants [19]. Studies and case reports are shown that implant placement after TDIs is a suitable treatment of choice [20–22].

In the epidemiological study, Ugolini et al. [1] determined the prevalence, types, and characteristics of occupational (work-related) TDIs in a large working community where among 212 traumatized teeth, upper incisors took the first place with 67.5%, lower incisors showed 17.5% incidence, upper canines were only 3.3%, lower canines with 1.9% were less than uppers, and bicuspids and molars had 9.9% prevalence. In conclusion occupational TDIs exhibit a low prevalence and the most frequent dental injury type were fractures. Possible etiologic risk factors for occupational TDIs were mentioned to be the age, gender and existence of previous dental treatments.

Rozi et al. [15] studied complications of permanents teeth after TDIs in 50 children [age range 7–18 years (mean, 11 years); 32 (64%) males and 18 (36%) females]. According to the findings of this study, TDIs mostly involved the maxillary central incisors by 90% incidence. Uncomplicated enamel and dentin fracture without pulp exposure was the most common type of TDI with 62%. Only 50% of the cases showed luxation type injuries. The urgent and proper timing in treatment was underlined and it was considered to be the primary important strategy to increase the prognosis.

Zaleckiene et al. [2] reviewed etiology, prevalence and possible outcomes of dental trauma. TDIs prevalence was found to be different among countries. TDIs are more prevalent in permanent than in primary dentition. Treatment strategies are directed to eliminate undesired consequences, but TDIs in the young patient is often complicated and can continue during the rest of his/her life.

Atabek et al. [16] examined epidemiological and dental data from TDIs to primary and permanent teeth during the period from 2005 to 2010. The study included 120 girls (35.3%) and 220 boys (64.7%) with an average age of 9 years. The maxillary central incisors were most commonly affected teeth with a prevalence of 66.24%. The main cause of TDIs was found to be the falls by 70.1% incidence. In primary dentition highest percentage of injuries were subluxations with 36.4% rate. In permanent dentition, uncomplicated crown fractures by 44.9% incidence were most frequent type of injury. In conclusion they stated that the prognosis of dental trauma cases varies depending on the time elapsed after the trauma before treatment started.

Zengin et al. [3] evaluated TDIs recorded using the World Health Organization classification modified by Andreasen et al. As the prevalence in a group of 5800 patient 255 had TDI (4.4%). TDIs were related mostly to the age group of 11–20 years. As gender distribution most affected were males (153 cases) and females got less injuries (102 cases). The main cause of traumatic injury was related to falls with 68.2% incidence, and generally trauma was taken place during outdoor activities by 56.1% prevalence. Upper central incisors took first place among the most frequently injured teeth with primary teeth injuries of 64.5% and permanent teeth injuries of 72.5%. Uncomplicated crown fracture was the most frequent type of TDI seen in both primary dentition with a percentage of 63% and permanent dentition with 47% incidence. In the population of the study, TDIs prevalence was considered to be low.

Unal et al. [17] through a retrospective study identified TDIs of 591 children (range 0–14 years, average age: 10.79 ± 2.06) referred to university hospital between years 2007 and 2012 in Sivas, Turkey. TDIs mostly occurred in the children of 12–14 years age group with 14% incidence. Dento-enamel fractures was the most common type of injury in primary teeth with 58% prevalence. Complicated crown fractures were most frequent type of TDI in permanent teeth with an incidence of 39%. The major etiologic factor of TDI was falls having 30% prevalence. The upper central incisors (71%) were the mostly affected teeth in both primary and permanent teeth. Only 63 children (11%) were referred to the clinic less than 30 minutes after trauma. The findings of this study showed that initial treatment after dental trauma should be performed immediately.

Kovacs et al. [4] in a retrospective study assessed the prevalence of TDIs in deciduous and permanent teeth among children and teenagers in Targu Mures city of Romania, between 2003 and 2011. The prevalence of TDIs was 24.5%. In the primary dentition the most frequent type of TDI was lateral incisor's luxation. In the permanent dentition, dento-enamel fractures without the exposure of the dental pulp were the most common type of TDI.

Hasan et al. [5] investigated a total of 500 of preschool children in Kuwait. The study reported TDIs etiologic factors, frequency, trauma type classification, injury localization and involved teeth numbers, treatment performed after injury. Among 500 children 56 subject got TDI involving 68 primary teeth with a prevalence of 11.2%. Fifty-three of 56 children got TDIs due to falls (94.6%). Upper primary central incisor was the most traumatized tooth with 55 units and 80.8% frequency. TDIs prevalence among such population was considered to be low.

Glendor [23] reviewed 12-years international literature regarding TDI to point the prevalence and incidence. TDIs were found to be a global phenomenon all over the world with variations in prevalence, etiologic factors, gender and localization of involved teeth. Across the world with slight differences from country to country, approximately 1/3 of preschool children got TDI in the primary dentition. Regarding TDI to the permanent dentition it could be concluded that although few variations among countries, about 1/4 of school children and almost 1/3 of adults received trauma.

According to Locker [13], 15.5% of the Canadians with age between 18 and 50 years old, living in the province of Ontario reported a history of injury to the mouth and teeth. The survey of this study involved 2001 adults who called by random digit dialing and answered to a questionnaire via telephone. Among the people who got TDI, 2/3 declared that injuries happened before the age of 18 years and 1/3 after adolescence.

Kaste et al. [14] reported findings of 7707 patients. According to Kaste's study, approximately one-quarter (24.9%) of the US population aged 6–50 years had at least one traumatized teeth.

Zerman and Cavalleri [6] examined 2798 patients having 6–21 years old age, with a follow-up period of 5-years in Verona, Italy. Among abovementioned population 178 were TDI cases, 131 males and 47 females, having 326 traumatized incisor teeth with a prevalence of 7.3%. Most frequent causes of injuries were falls and traffic accidents. A very large number of dental injuries occurred to children aged between 6 and 13 years. Most injuries involved two teeth. About 80% of the teeth were maxillary central incisors.

3. Dental implant treatment in post-traumatic dento-alveolar defects

In the literature there are numerous case reports and few clinical studies documenting treatment options of post-trauma patients by dental implants [24–29]. In those reports and studies cases underwent to trauma due to violence, falls, traffic injuries, gunshots which were later rehabilitated by use of dental implants are described in details. Treatment approaches reported are various as the cases exhibit different conditions related to the type of trauma, anatomy and age. Principally there are some limitations of dental implant application related to the age and available bone volume of patients. One of the main criteria for dental implant placement is the presence of complete bone growth as the metallic implants do not follow bony development phases [30–34]. Most often TDIs occur in childhood and implant treatment should postponed as mentioned [31]. Thus, the children who receives TDIs should wear removable or adhesive prosthesis until their skeleton mature. In this aspect the major problem associated with dental implant placement is the lack of adequate bone volumes at the future time of surgery as such cases receives TDI in the early years and disuse atrophy occurs during waiting period [21]. Maxillary central incisors area which is commonly affected zone by TDIs is most apparent site of the dentition and requires proper dimensions and proportions to establish esthetic and require complex treatment solutions such as bone grafting with autogenous or synthetic graft materials, guided bone regeneration applications; immediate, early or delayed implant placement methods (**Figures 1**–7).

Nicoli et al. [24] wrote records of a multidisciplinary treatment made in a gunshot injury case. Patient got severe anatomic defect in the mandible which was rehabilitated by use of an implant-supported fixed-removable dental prosthesis. In order to restore intermaxillary relation an immediately loaded provisional lower overdenture and upper removable prosthesis were delivered.

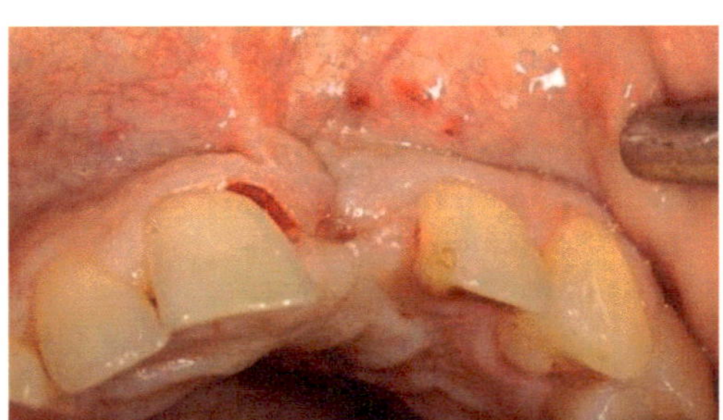

Figure 1.
Traffic accident case: central incisor number 21 was lost due to a traffic incident trauma; bone volüme was reduced in the buccal side and soft tissue was injured by a vertical laceration in the medial part of keratinized mucosa.

Following interim prosthesis installations, in order to increase the maxillary bone volume, nasal floor elevation and maxillary sinus lifting operations were performed. Subsequently definitive implant-supported fixed-removable prostheses were delivered in both arches to improve masticatory function and esthetics.

Fındık et al. [25] presented rehabilitation of a wide mandibular traumatic defect due to a work-related accident with iliac free flap, distraction osteogenesis, and dental implants. Distraction osteogenesis, free flap and dental implant placements were considered as an effective and esthetic treatment option for rehabilitation of post-trauma defects.

Balla et al. [26] described 5-year follow-up of surgical and prosthetic reconstruction of a gunshot injury using dental implants which was found to be

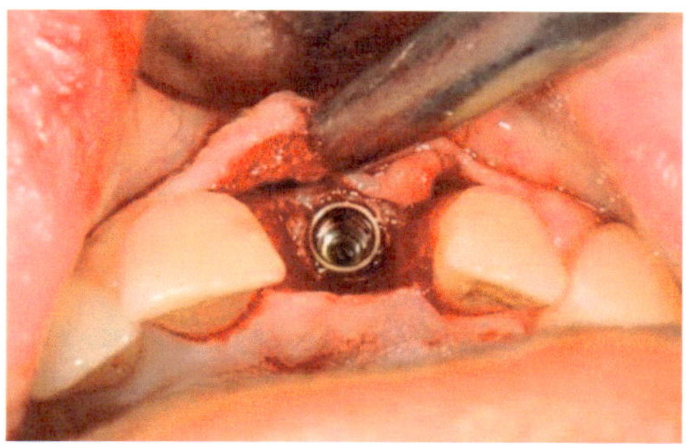

Figure 2.
Titanium/zirconia alloy dental implant (Bone Level SLA, Straumann AG, Swiss) was placed.

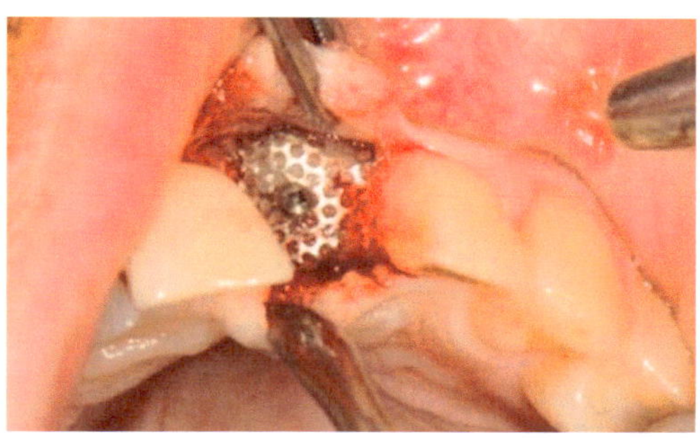

Figure 3.
Titanium mesh was placed on the buccal side and secured into the implant by cover screw.

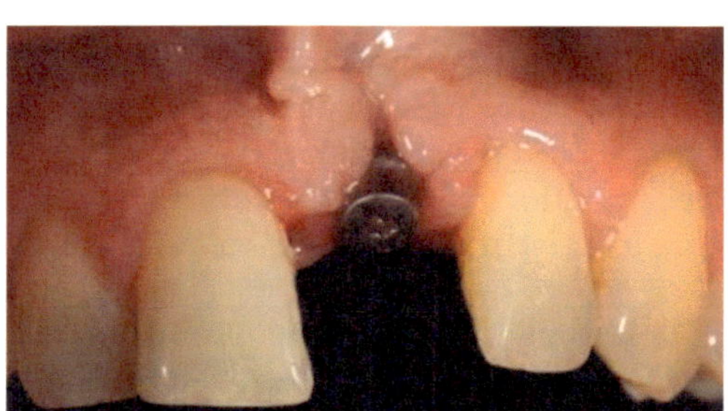

Figure 4.
After 6 weeks of healing period a mucosa former abutment was placed. The laceratio formed after traffic accident still persist on the buccal mucosa.

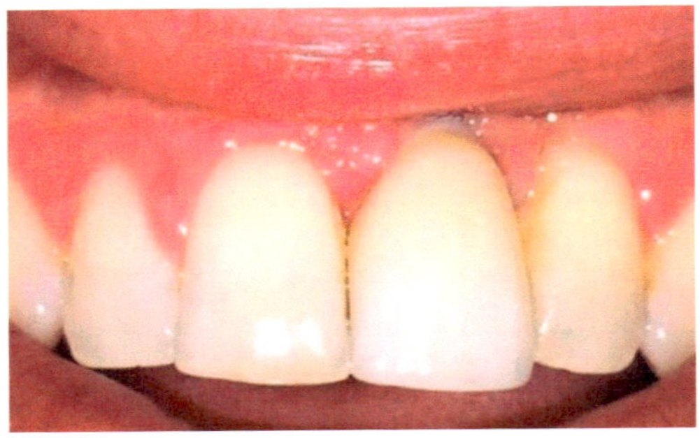

Figure 5.
Intraoral appearance of implant supported lithium disilicate single crown placed on top of custon zirconia abutment.

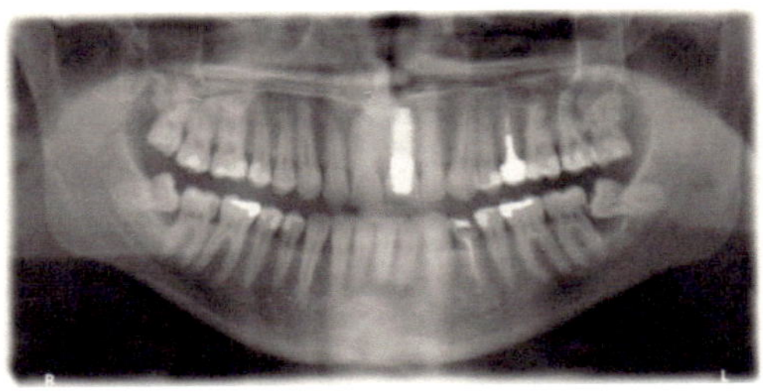

Figure 6.
OPG after crown placement.

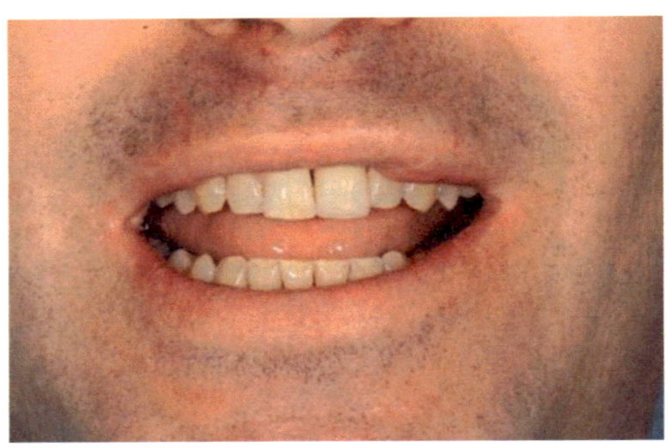

Figure 7.
Appearance after prosthesis delivery: note hypertrophic sequelae of upper left lip due to traffic accident.

effective treatment modality in restoring a patient to near normal function and esthetics. According to this study, maxillofacial injuries made by gunshot create serious esthetic, functional, and psychological consequences. Disabling characteristic of such severe maxillofacial ballistic defects brings the need of challenging extensive reconstructive multiple surgeries and competitive prosthetic rehabilitation phases.

Jain and Baliga [27] described two cases with maxillofacial trauma and had undergone open reduction and internal fixation where implant placement was done for upper anterior teeth.

Sharma and Swamy [28] reported a gunshot case who lost six teeth in maxilla and was rehabilitated by rotated flap, bone grafts and three dental implants supporting a FPD.

Wang et al. [29] mentioned the treatment a 17-year-old boy having maxillofacial ballistic defects. They described multiple techniques for restoration of facial morphology and function. Multiple examinations and surgical procedures including osteomyocutaneous and muscular flaps in combination with dental implants were used to restore facial morphology, functions of mastication and articulation.

Generally implant placement is planned after orthodontic treatment to gain adequate space [21]. But there are exceptions reported depending from the needs and anatomy of individuals such as Kuo et al. [35] who reported a case where after a traumatic loss of upper incisor an implant was placed and subsequent orthodontic treatment was performed.

Kulkarni et al. [36] reported ballistic injury of a 24-year-old man. Maxillofacial deficiency was restored with autogenous iliac bone graft. Following 3 months of healing dental implants were placed. After osseointegration period of 5 months fixed-removable hybrid prosthesis was installed. At the end of third year of hybrid prosthesis usage, it was renewed by a porcelain fused to metal bridge. Follow-up on radiographies showed that the crestal bone levels around implants were stable. Kulkarni et al. [36] stated that the rehabilitation of gunshot injuries is expanded within time and needs several interventions to obtain functional and esthetics requirements.

Seymour et al. [37] mentioned the need of team approach in the rehabilitation severe trauma cases and underlined the importance of communication between general practitioners and specialist especially in the complex dental implant treatments.

Chesterman et al. [38] described guidelines regarding the replacement of single teeth lost due to trauma with implant supported restorations. The protocol proposed includes: evaluation of tooth replacement methods; planning for tooth loss and provision of an implant supported restoration; planning of an implant supported restoration.

Alani et al. [39] stated that with advances in both adhesive technologies and implant dentistry, there are a variety of options for the restoration of edentulism subsequent to TDIs.

Pae et al. [22] described a panfacial fracture case who was managed with a mandibular implant-supported fixed-removable and a maxillary partial removable prosthesis where due to the lack of intraoral landmarks, overall facial anatomic landmarks were used to restore the oral cavity.

Kamoi [40] reported treatment history of a 44-year-old woman who had severe injuries due to traffic accident. The patient got maxillofacial soft tissue lacerations followed by hard tissue fractures, several teeth loss associated with alveolar bone resorption. Several facial reconstructions were made by plastic surgeons. To replace missing upper teeth a sinus grafting procedure was performed by use of a rib bone anchorage and simultaneous placement of five dental implants. After 11 months of healing period, upper overdenture and a mandibular PFM's were fabricated. The outcome of the treatment was found to be satisfactory.

Robinson and Cunningham [41] described the oral rehabilitation of an adult male who suffered severe dentoalveolar trauma as a result of a motor vehicle accident. After extraction of fractured roots, dental implants were placed. Following certain healing period for osseointegration, PFM crowns and FPD's were installed. In a 3-year follow-up period, the outcomes of the treatment were considered to be successful regarding patient's esthetic and functional expectations.

Schneider et al. [42] reported the surgical and prosthodontic rehabilitation of a patient traumatized by a self-inflicted gunshot wound to the mandible which required rehabilitation with a free fibula microvascular graft, single stage dental implant placement, and rehabilitation with CAD/CAM and laser assembled prosthetic components.

Nissan et al. [43] evaluated the outcome of dental implants placed in the post-traumatic anterior maxilla after ridge augmentation with cancellous freeze-dried block bone allografts. After 6 months of healing, implants were placed. The study group was composed of 20 consecutive patients with a mean age of 25 ± 7 years, received 31 implants, 12 of them were immediately restored. Graft and implant survival rates were 92.8 and 96.8%, respectively. There were no changes in bone to implant contact (BIC) levels. The authors considered predictable the usage of cancellous block allografts in the reconstruction of post-traumatic defects of anterior maxilla.

Yamano et al. [44] gave treatment history of a 15-year-old male patient who had a snowmobile accident. Patient got maxillofacial defects and fractures in mid-face and mandible. A multidisciplinary rehabilitation was performed to restore function and esthetics. Treatments involved usage of autologous corticocancellous bone grafts, fixture placement and implant-supported prosthesis fabrication.

A ballistic maxillofacial injury case and her treatment modality was described by Torabi et al. [45] The patient received trauma in maxilla, mandible and nasal areas with heavy problems in her esthetics and functions. Dental implants were used in conjunction with natural abutments to restore dentition.

Bird and Veeranki [46] reported a maxillofacial ballistic injury case rehabilitated with iliac crest bone graft, dental implants, and an economical acrylic resin fixed prosthesis. A 3-year follow-up revealed positive treatment outcomes and it was concluded that although facial gunshots cause severe defects, they can be restored and rehabilitated by a multidisciplinary approach. They outlined the importance of and biomechanical considerations for implant positioning.

Kelly and Drago [12] described a patient who suffered significant trauma to the lower and mid-face secondary to a gunshot injury. The size and severity of the defects are in proportion with the functional and esthetic complications faced during the late phases of the treatment. Regardless to the amount of facial trauma, successful treatment can be performed by appropriate clinical and radiographic examinations and diagnosis followed with correct treatment strategies and applications strictly linked to surgical and prosthodontic principles.

Gökçen-Röhlig et al. [47] described the rehabilitation of a patient with a mandibular defect caused by a gunshot wound who was treated with four osseointegrated implant-supported mandibular overdenture and maxillary removable prosthesis. Despite anatomic limitations, the patient's esthetic and functional demands were fulfilled.

Sándor and Carmichael [48] proposed to respect growth and delay implant reconstruction until the cessation of skeletal or alveolar growth.

In the 2-year follow-up report of a traffic accident and traumatic injury happen to 16 years old male patient who was rehabilitated by autogenous graft and four dental implants, outcomes were found to be satisfactory and stable [49].

Sipahi et al. [50] reported a self-inflicted gunshot maxillofacial defect case who was restored with dental implants and various prosthetic attachments. During short-term follow-up period no complications were occurred. The outcome of a fixed-removable implant-supported mandibular prosthesis and a maxillary obturator was considered successful in the management of a serious traumatic injury.

Clinical evaluation of a mandibular ballistic injury patient was described by Cakan et al. [51]. The patient was treated with cemented crowns for 2 maxillary implants and an implant-supported screw-retained fixed partial denture supported by eight mandibular implants. Although difficulties to properly position the implants because of inadequate bone volume, esthetic and functional demands of the patient were fulfilled.

Schwartz-Arad and Levin [20] examined a patient pool of 53 individuals having dental implants after traumatic injury history in the anterior maxilla. They found significantly lower complications in the group of patients which did not have inflammatory lesions in their history. Meanwhile patients who lost their teeth due to inflammatory lesions after traumatic injuries got statistically significant amount of complications and failures with dental implants. They underlined the necessity for scrupulous diagnosis of teeth and alveolar bone after a traumatic injury in order to reduce complications and advised individualized treatment planning for each case as the methodology is multidisciplinary.

Schwartz-Arad et al. [21] mentioned the difficulties in the dental implant based rehabilitations in patients who got traumatic injuries in childhood where implant placement is contraindicated during growth period and on the other hand they need replacement of missing teeth and also preserve adequate jaw bone volume for future implant placement. Various treatment strategies were suggested until the end of growth and development. Among them, orthodontic extrusion of the root fragment and a temporary crown application technique in order to preserve alveolar bone, autogenous tooth transplantation, intentional extraction and immediate tooth replantation, distraction osteogenesis, and decoronation could be mentioned.

Five-year follow-up results of 42 single-tooth implant treatment in 34 trauma-related edentulous patients were evaluated by Andersson et al. [52]. In this patient pool the most frequently lost teeth were upper central incisors with an incidence of 75%. In the second place there were lateral incisors with 21% frequency. In growing patients, implant treatment was generally postponed until completion of development. Preservation of roots in the alveolar process seemed to maintain the bone volume enabling better conditions for later implant placement. According to the findings of this study, the functional and esthetic outcome of single-tooth implant treatment can be recommended for replacing tooth losses after trauma in the anterior region of the maxilla.

Tipton [53] reported a case who had TDI due to an accident and rehabilitation protocol with a team approach for dental implant restoration. The outcome was considered excellent regarding the teamwork among the dentist, implant surgeon, and laboratory technician following traumatic injury of the dentition.

4. Prerequisites for dental implant placement after trauma

Systemic conditions and history of the patient should be favorable to the surgery. In the medical history of the patient possible genetic, autoimmune and connective tissue diseases must be investigated in order to reduce risk factors [54]. In the history of patient presence of recent cerebrovascular disturbance and myocardial infarct, ongoing immunosuppressive [55] or chemotherapy, fibrous dysplasia [56–58], intravenous bisphosphonate therapies [59–64], uncontrolled diabetes [65–69], narcotic dependencies or psychiatric diseases form absolute contraindication for dental implant treatment [70]. In such conditions alternative prosthodontic treatments should be planned. Some form of diseases, treatments and drug therapies which affect metabolic activity of body and habits are considered to be relative contraindications as they reduce success and longevity of osseointegration. In the presence of any relative contraindication it must be evaluated the need of dental implant treatment for the patient and health conditions in the decision-making phase. Among relative contraindications there are past radiotherapies with irradiated jawbones [71–74], diabetes, autoimmune connective tissue diseases (rheumatoid arthritis [75–77], Sjögren's syndrome [78], Lupus Erythematosus [79], Papillon-Lefevre syndrome [80–82], Behcet disease, Myasthenia Gravis, Ectodermal Dysplasia [83–87], Skeleroderma [88–90]), calcium-phosphate metabolism disorders and endocrine diseases (osteoporosis, osteopenia, Paget disease, hyper and hypothyroidism, kidney nephritis, aldosteronism, Cushing syndrome), viral diseases (HIV, Hepatitis III), aggressive periodontitis, smoking, drug abuse, oral bisphosphonate usage, unstable psychological state. Other risk factors which should be evaluated during treatment planning are parafunctions-bruxism and facial dystonia [91].

Animal model studies have shown that metallic implants do not change location in concordance with three-dimensional bony growth [92–95]. Dental implants do not follow bone development during growth period [34, 92–101]. Studies have shown that implants placed in the early ages remain in infra-occlusion by time [99]. For this reason as the consensus, implant treatment is made after confirming bony development period of patient by hand-wrist radiographies and comparisons in radiography-skeleton atlas [98, 100]. Ulnar sesamoid cartilage and middle finger's middle phalanx distal cartilage ossification rate is inspected and compared with images in skeleton atlas. For the minimal age of implant surgery decision instead of chronological age, skeletal age of patient is taken in consideration. Patients who are within the active bone growth period can receive removable prosthesis or adhesive prosthesis. In children adhesive prosthesis such as Maryland type are splinting teeth together and apply stationery anchorage against three-dimensional enlargement of jawbones during active bone growth. Growing patients should periodically controlled and adhesive prosthesis should modify in case of need. In future implant placement plans traumatized roots should be kept in place as space maintainers although their prognosis is poor. Slow orthodontic extrusion of traumatized hopeless roots is one of the bone guidance methods in order to create adequate hard tissue volume for upcoming dental implant rehabilitation [102].

The first prerequisite in implant dentistry is the presence of adequate vital bone volume to entirely cover the implant body [103]. If trauma happens in childhood ending with tooth loose, patient should wait certain years until active bone growth completes before implant placement and during waiting period bone volume decrease in edentulous areas by disuse atrophy. In atrophic crests various augmentation method could be applied. The first choice of augmentation material is autogenous bone grafts. Autogenous bone graft blocks can be placed over recipient residual bone site and fixed by mini-screws, or 'Bone Lamina' technique which consist in splitting a bone block in thin layers and fix them onto the augmentation area by mini-screws as shields to create a certain volume and fill inside the shields with particulate autogenous or synthetic grafts. Autogenous bone grafts are always considered as the golden standard in augmentation procedures. Secondly osteoconductive ceramic alloplast (hydroxylapatite, tricalcium phosphate) or xenografts (bovine, mini-pig, single-hoofed) are preferred. Demineralized, demineralized freeze-dried or frozen homolog transplants although are osteoinductive they have non-predictable life-time and may not be adequate to complete osteogenesis phases in time scale. Other augmentation alternative is the usage of titanium grid-mesh (Ti-mesh) shields to obtain tent effect and fulfill them by particulated graft materials. Similarly, Guided Bone Regeneration (GBR) technique can be applied by use of resorbable or non-resorbable membranes alone or in conjunction with graft materials according to the defect size. Split-bone technique is suitable for crests thicker than 3 mm in buccopalatal section and mainly is adequate for pliable maxilla rather than less elastic mandible. Crestal bone is splinted in equal two pieces by micro-saws, piezoelectric inserts or Erbium Yttrium Aluminum Garnet (Er:YAG) laser until bypassing cortical bone. Once spongious bone is arrived special splitter osteotome inserts are placed into osteotomy site. To avoid unpredictable fractures vertical release osteotomies should be made in the extremities of the working field. Distraction osteogenesis is another technique well documented for bone augmentation. But distraction appliances are difficult to maintain for children in the interactive play age and could be further traumatized often.

The choice of augmentation method depends on the defect size, volume, tridimensional shape of hard tissues and biotype of soft tissues. If the vertical dimension of the crest is normal but bucco-palatal width is missing GBR, Ti-mesh, Split-bone, onlay graft, Bone Lamina techniques could be used. When the vertical bone height is lost onlay grafting, Bone Lamina, distraction osteogenesis and Ti-mesh would be preferences. Soft tissue thickness establishes biotype of mucosa. Thin biotypes are difficult to manage as they are fragile and difficult elongate in order to achieve tension free flap. Flaps which cover wound should be overlay on grafted area without pressure in order to obtain normal blood supply. If there would be several tensions on the flap, vascular network will suffer and due to the lack of nutrition surgery can fail. Flap design gain certain importance to have profuse blood circulation. Flaps with larger base than free edge, possibly without vertical release incisions can maintain vascular network without interruption of capillary arteriae and vessels. Anatomic studies have shown that within the buccal and palatal mucosa, capillary networks do not constitute anastomosis on the top crestal region of maxilla and mandible [104]. Thus by mid-crestal incisions there is no interruption of vessels and this type of incision should be choice of preference. Mucosal flaps according to depth could be 'full-thickness' where epithelium, connective tissue and underlying periosteum are excited and elevated together; or 'split-thickness' where periosteum is left attached to the cortical bone to avoid blood supply interruption (because capillary arteriae network is situated within the periosteum and 70% nutrition of the cortical bone derives from periosteum), and to have elasticity of the flap (periosteum do not have elastic behavior). Thick biotype mucosa has an advantage in terms of elongation. To elongate a full-thickness flap the basal portion of it which is constituted by periosteum should be gently incited horizontally. In such manner the rigidity of the periosteum is alternated and underlying connective tissue portion would elongate easily as contains elastin fibers of collagen. Split-thickness flaps could be preferred only in thick biotype mucosa as the thin biotype is difficult to split and fragile.

Implant's primary stability is another prerequisite to achieve osseointegration. Studies have shown that dental implants can integrate with surrounding bone if they have less than 100 microstrain or less than 150 micron micromovement [105–109]. Early loading of dental implants do not interfere with surrounding bone mineral apposition speed and osteogenesis phases continues to integrate with implant surface if primary stability is achieved [105–111]. Osteoblast phenotype morphology and physiology are not altered in immediately or early loaded implants [108, 110]. Adequate primary stability for a dental implant could be interpreted by insertion torque values greater than 30 N/cm^2. Primary stability and in the following time period stability of implants could be measured by use of Resonance Frequency Analysis (RFA) method [112–114]. RFA works by vibrations transmitted to implant body and measurement of implant's resistance values in numbers expressed in Implant Stability Quotient (ISQ) units. Studies conducted with RFA showed that peri-implant bone strength follows Normal Distribution Curve (bell curve) as seen in many natural phenomena. Initial strength of interfacial bone to the implant due to inflammatory reactions and acidic environment decreases and reach the weakest point in the third week after implant placement. Meanwhile mineral apposition and developing ossification take place and secondary stability increase after third week to reach initial stability ISQ values approximately in the sixth week. The studies made on micro-movement and micro-strain have shown the possibility of osseointegration in immediate loading situation unless the threshold of 100 micron of mobility is not exceed [105–107]. Based on such results, it has been introduced 'immediate loading' protocol by use of splinted implants for totally edentulous patients [106, 109]. There are promising results and developing protocols of immediate loading for partially edentulous and missing single-tooth cases, where the requirements are presence of primary stability more than 30 N/cm^2, implant length more than 10 mm, implant diameter more than 3.75 mm for titanium or zirconia dental implants and 3.3 mm for titanium-zirconia alloy implants, rigid splint of implants (in partially edentulous cases), non-functional loading, temporization (immediate delivery of provisional crowns or bridges to shape soft tissue contours). In patients where there are short implants but adequate primary stability, or patients with parafunctions, patients with low density bone (type III or IV), 'early loading' protocol which previews 6 weeks healing period can be applied. If the primary stability of an implant is less than 30 N/cm^2 insertion torque, healing period should be elongated to 3 months for the lower and 6 months for the upper jaw bones which is called 'delayed loading' protocol as proposed by Branemark at the beginning years of modern scientific implant dentistry.

TDI cases mostly involve anterior maxilla with early or delayed loss of single tooth (except gunshots) which is mainly central incisor. In single-tooth replacements there are special rules to follow in order to obtain suitable esthetics. Maintenance of soft tissue envelope contours and the presence of papillae are highly important. The preservation of soft tissue integrity is related to flap nutrition, thus flapless surgery is the primary choice. The 'tunnel technique' may be an alternative to conventional open flap surgery and graft application, in order to apply minimally invasive surgery. Another approach is to avoid vertical release incisions and apply only sulcular incision to keep intact vessels of flap and cause less reduction of blood supply.

Papilla protective flap design is thought to preserve papillae, where two vertical incisions exclude papillae in both distal and mesial sides and a narrow full thickness flap band is raised. In long term follow-ups it has been noted that those two vertical incisions lead the formation of scar areas which would apparent on the buccal side of mucosa. On the other hand, in case of intra-operative treatment plan change, upon need of augmentation, the graft materials would be under incision lines. The presence of incisions on the grafted area will increase microbial contamination risk of graft by micro-leakage and cause inadequate blood supply to the graft. Thus, papilla protective flap design is almost a disappeared technique.

The second rule to follow in single-tooth replacements is the preservation of buccal bony wall. In jaw bones anatomy, buccal portion of alveolar bones is mostly very thin [115–117]. This thin buccal wall would be resorbed rapidly due to acidic inflammatory environment which may take place in case of nutrition lack due to flap raising, or after trauma and post-traumatic extraction where crestal bone could be fractured. To avoid traumatic extractions periotomes, electro-dynamomagnetic device inserts, piezoelectric device inserts, special extraction drill-chain appliances, very thin Er:YAG laser sapphire tips are developed. 'Ridge preservation' techniques which aims to immediately graft extraction sockets to avoid future resorptions are proposed. Some authors proposed not only hard tissue grafting but also mucosa transplants by punch technique to cover entirely socket orifice. On the horizontal plane palato-position of the implant placement is another rule to follow to preserve buccal width of alveolar bone. Palato-position of an implant is obtained by centering the insertion point of first drills on the palatal wall of the socket, but not to the apical bottom; the location should be slightly palatal to the inter-incisal line of adjacent teeth. Plato-positioning helps also to balance the future unavoidable senile resoption pattern of buccal alveolar bones which is physiological. A single-tooth implant should keep equal distance to the neighboring teeth. The collar platform level of the single-tooth implant should not be embedded more than 2 mm apically from the cementoenamel junction (CEJ) of adjacent teeth. If the implant collar exceeds CEJ criteria, longest crowns in comparison to natural dentition should be fabricated and the future bacterial colonization of inner implant spaces will execute pumping effect of contaminants deriving from the micro-gaps between abutment-implant connection during chewing cycles which will result in collar area bone resorption and subsequent mucosal recessions and papilla loosening.

In adolescent patients who completed their skeletal growth and in adults after traumatic loss of teeth if the available soft tissue and bone volumes are favorable, implants could be placed immediately. Immediate implant placement may be excluded when the soft tissues have lost their integrity to cover wound area by tension-free flaps; or when hard tissues have great volume loss and primary anchorage possibility would poor (e.g., traffic accidents, gunshots). In such situations primary wound healing should be waited. The risk in immediate implant placement after trauma is associated with the contamination of defect area by foreign bodies and microorganisms. To clean extraction socket generally conventional curettage is followed. But bacterial contamination can still persist within the lamina cribrosa of socket or in the spongy bone. The best method to avoid contaminants and bacteria from the wound area would be usage of Er:YAG laser irradiation associated with conventional curettage as the studies have shown Er:YAG's high bactericidal effect against microbiota [118–120].

In the anterior region of jaws titanium implant body and abutment reflection may be apparent by time as buccal bone senile resorption pattern is from distal (outside) to medial (inside). Solution to mask metallic reflection is the usage of ceramic materials. Recently full ceramic zirconia implants and abutments gained again popularity. After first attempts of alumina implants in the 1970s and their mechanic failures caused an interval of approximately 30 years. In last two decades, firstly CAD/CAM zirconia abutments and following one-piece zirconia and recently two-pieces zirconia implants were introduced in the market. Nowadays most sophisticated applications of single-tooth replacements are made by full ceramic implants, zirconia-titanium or titanium implants and zirconia abutments supporting leucite-reinforced ceramic or lithium disilicate ceramic crowns.

Future trends and strategies in dental traumatology in general and with special attention to dental implant applications are based on the education of population in terms of emergency treatments and urgent transport of patients to the clinics; trained clinics on emergency treatments; preparation of patients to future implant rehabilitations by interim treatment which care preservation of hard and soft tissues.

5. Conclusions

Edentulism due to trauma could be properly rehabilitated by dental implant placements. Reports in the literature have been adequately evidenced safe usage of dental implants after traumatic injuries. There are various considerations to plan suitable treatment option in the edentulous areas of jawbones after trauma. At the first side the systemic conditions of patient should permit dental implant surgery. Secondly the skeletal age of patient should be adequate to implant placement as it is shown that implants do not migrate following bony development and embed in an infra-occlusion by time. The third level of consideration is the availability of soft and hard tissues. Rehabilitation strategies are developed according to the defect size, volume, tridimensional shape of hard tissues and biotype of soft tissues. Special attention is paid to preserve mucosal contours and papillae by use of flapless technique or proper incisions, as well as hard tissue augmentation options are planned taking in consideration the available vascularity, defect wall number, bone height and fixation of graft material. In the implant placement phase the primary stability is the main target in order to initiate osseointegration. There are several implant insertion techniques such as drilling, narrow drill/wider implant, osteotome, bone splint and laser-assisted which are decided basing on possible primary anchorage within the residual bone. After achievement of primary stability it should be decided the loading type of implants which is related to implant number, localization, length, diameter, splinting options. Basically functional immediate, non-functional immediate, early or delayed loading protocols can be applied. Once loading protocol is fixed it should be emphasized the prosthetic supra-structure design and material. In conclusion missing teeth due to trauma could be successfully rehabilitated by dental implants following detailed and careful diagnosis in order to establish proper individual treatment plan and by application of consecutive treatment steps.

Author details

Tosun Tosun[1]* and Koray Meltem[2]

1 Department of Oral and Maxillofacial Surgery, Dental School, Istanbul Aydin University, Istanbul, Turkey

2 Department of Oral and Maxillofacial Surgery, Dental School, Istanbul University, Istanbul, Turkey

*Address all correspondence to: tosuntosun@aydin.edu.tr

References

[1] Ugolini A, Parodi GB, Casali C, Silvestrini-Biavati A, Giacinti F. Work-related traumatic dental injuries: Prevalence, characteristics and risk factors. Dental Traumatology. 2018;**34**(1):36-40

[2] Zaleckiene V, Peciuliene V, Brukiene V, Drukteinis S. Traumatic dental injuries: Etiology, prevalence and possible outcomes. Stomatologija. 2014;**16**(1):7-14

[3] Zengin AZ, Celenk P, Sumer AP, Cankaya S. Evaluation of traumatic dental injuries in a group of Turkish population. Nigerian Journal of Clinical Practice. 2015;**18**(1):86-89

[4] Kovacs M, Pacurar M, Petcu B, Bukhari C. Prevalence of traumatic dental injuries in children who attended two dental clinics in Targu Mures between 2003 and 2011. Oral Health and Dental Management. 2012;**11**(3):116-124

[5] Hasan AA, Qudeimat MA, Andersson L. Prevalence of traumatic dental injuries in preschool children in Kuwait - a screening study. Dental Traumatology. 2010;**26**(4):346-350

[6] Zerman N, Cavalleri G. Traumatic injuries to permanent incisors. Endodontics & Dental Traumatology. 1993;**9**(2):61-64

[7] Andersson L. Epidemiology of traumatic dental injuries. Journal of Endodontia. 2013;**39**(3 Suppl):S2-S5

[8] Andreasen JO, Lauridsen E. Alveolar process fractures in the permanent dentition. Part 1. Etiology and clinical characteristics. A retrospective analysis of 299 cases involving 815 teeth. Dental Traumatology. 2015;**31**(6):442-447

[9] Diangelis AJ et al. International Association of Dental Traumatology guidelines for the management of traumatic dental injuries: 1. Fractures and luxations of permanent teeth. Dental Traumatology. 2012;**28**(1):2-12

[10] Malmgren B et al. International Association of Dental Traumatology guidelines for the management of traumatic dental injuries: 3. Injuries in the primary dentition. Dental Traumatology. 2013;**28**(3):174-182

[11] Vatsyayan A, Adhyapok A-K, Debnath S-C, Malik K. Reconstruction and rehabilitation of short-range gunshot injury to lower part of face: A systematic approach of three cases. Chinese Journal of Traumatology = Zhonghua chuang shang za zhi. 2016;**19**(4):239-243

[12] Kelly P, Drago CJ. Surgical and prosthodontic treatment of a patient with significant trauma to the middle and lower face secondary to a gunshot wound: A clinical report. Journal of Prosthodontics. 2009;**18**(7):626-637

[13] Locker D. Self-reported dental and oral injuries in a population of adults aged 18-50 years. Dental Traumatology. 2007;**23**(5):291-296

[14] Kaste LM, Gift HC, Bhat M, Swango PA. Prevalence of incisor trauma in persons 6-50 years of age: United States, 1988-1991. Journal of Dental Research. 1996;**75**(Spec. Issue):696-705

[15] Rozi AH, Scott JM, Seminario AL. Trauma in permanent teeth: Factors associated with adverse outcomes in a university pediatric dental clinic. Journal of Dentistry for Children (Chicago, IL.). 2017;**84**(1):9-15

[16] Atabek D, Alaçam A, Aydintuğ I, Konakoğlu G. A retrospective study of traumatic dental injuries. Dental Traumatology. 2014;**30**(2):154-161

[17] Unal M, Oznurhan F, Kapdan A, Aksoy S, Dürer A. Traumatic dental

injuries in children. Experience of a hospital in the central Anatolia region of Turkey. European Journal of Paediatric Dentistry. 2014;**15**(1):17-22

[18] Andersson L et al. International Association of Dental Traumatology guidelines for the management of traumatic dental injuries: 2. Avulsion of permanent teeth. Dental Traumatology. 2012;**28**(2):88-96

[19] Cvek M, Tsilingaridis G, Andreasen JO. Survival of 534 incisors after intra-alveolar root fracture in patients aged 7-17 years. Dental Traumatology. 2008;**24**(4):379-387

[20] Schwartz-Arad D, Levin L. Post-traumatic use of dental implants to rehabilitate anterior maxillary teeth. Dental Traumatology. 2004;**20**(6):344-347

[21] Schwartz-Arad D, Levin L, Ashkenazi M. Treatment options of untreatable traumatized anterior maxillary teeth for future use of dental implantation. Implant Dentistry. 2004;**13**(2):120-128

[22] Pae A, Choi C-H, Noh K, Kwon Y-D, Kim H-S, Kwon K-R. The prosthetic rehabilitation of a panfacial fracture patient after reduction: A clinical report. The Journal of Prosthetic Dentistry. 2012;**108**(2):123-128

[23] Glendor U. Epidemiology of traumatic dental injuries—A 12 year review of the literature. Dental Traumatology. 2008;**24**(6):603-611

[24] Nícoli LG, Pigossi SC, Araújo RF d SB, Marcantonio C, Marcantonio É, Marcantonio É. Multidisciplinary approach to oral rehabilitation with dental implants after gunshot injury: A clinical report. Journal of Prosthetic Dentistry. 2018;**119**(3):329-333

[25] Findik Y, Baykul T, Aydin MA, Altuntaş S, Demirekin ZB. Rehabilitation of the work accident-related traumatic mandible with iliac free flap, distraction osteogenesis, and dental implants. The Journal of Craniofacial Surgery. 2017;**28**(3):e238-e239

[26] Balla V, Daniel AY, Kurian N. Prosthodontic rehabilitation of accidental maxillofacial gunshot injury using dental implants: A five year follow-up clinical report. Journal of Clinical and Diagnostic Research. 2016;**10**(9):ZD06-ZD08

[27] Jain A, Baliga S. Rehabilitation of avulsed teeth in fractured jaws via bone grafting and implant placement: Report of two cases. Journal of Dentistry (Tehran). 2015;**12**(7):542-549

[28] Sharma MC, Swamy MM. Rehabilitation of a gunshot wound with dental implants. Medical Journal Armed Forces India. 2015;**71** (1 Suppl):S160-S162

[29] Wang W, Duan J, Wang Q, Kuang W. Complex reconstruction of facial deformity and function after severe gunshot injury: One case report. International Journal of Clinical and Experimental Medicine. 2015;**8**(1):1427-1433

[30] Mankani N, Chowdhary R, Patil BA, Nagaraj E, Madalli P. Osseointegrated Dental Implants in Growing Children: A Literature Review. The Journal of Oral Implantology. 2014;**40**(5):627-631

[31] Heij DGO, Opdebeeck H, van Steenberghe D, Kokich VG, Belser U, Quirynen M. Facial development, continuous tooth eruption, and mesial drift as compromising factors for implant placement. The International Journal of Oral & Maxillofacial Implants. 2006;**21**(6):867-878

[32] Bernard JP, Schatz JP, Christou P, Belser U, Kiliaridis S. Long-term vertical

changes of the anterior maxillary teeth adjacent to single implants in young and mature adults. A retrospective study. Journal of Clinical Periodontology. 2004;**31**(11):1024-1028

[33] Percinoto C, Vieira AE, Barbieri CM, Melhado FL, Moreira KS. Use of dental implants in children: A literature review. Quintessence International. 2001;**32**(5):381-383

[34] Thilander B, Odman J, Lekholm U. Orthodontic aspects of the use of oral implants in adolescents: A 10-year follow-up study. European Journal of Orthodontics. 2001;**23**(6):715-731

[35] Kuo T-J, Chang H-J, Hsieh Y-D, Wu C-N, Chen C-C. An alternative approach sequence to early implant placement and bone grafting over upper incisor traumatic loss in a malocclusion patient. The Journal of Oral Implantology. 2015;**41**(2):214-218

[36] Kulkarni S et al. Rehabilitation of a patient with gunshot injury through the iliac graft and implant-retained restorations with a 3-year follow-up: A brief clinical study. The Journal of Craniofacial Surgery. 2014;**25**(2):e207-e210

[37] Seymour DW, Patel M, Carter L, Chan M. The management of traumatic tooth loss with dental implants: Part 2. Severe trauma. British Dental Journal. 2014;**217**(12):667-671

[38] Chesterman J, Chauhan R, Patel M, Chan MFW-Y. The management of traumatic tooth loss with dental implants: Part 1. British Dental Journal. 2014;**217**(11):627-633

[39] Alani A, Austin R, Djemal S. Contemporary management of tooth replacement in the traumatized dentition. Dental Traumatology. 2012;**28**(3):183-192

[40] Kamoi H. A case of recovery of oral function with dental implants following facial bone trauma. Journal of Nippon Medical School. 2012;**79**(6):484-488

[41] Robinson FG, Cunningham LL. Oral rehabilitation of severe dentoalveolar trauma: A clinical report. The Journal of Oral Implantology. 2012;**38**(6):757-761

[42] Schneider R, Fridrich K, Chang K. Complex mandibular rehabilitation of a self-inflicted gunshot wound: A clinical report. The Journal of Prosthetic Dentistry. 2012;**107**(3):158-162

[43] Nissan J, Gross O, Mardinger O, Ghelfan O, Sacco R, Chaushu G. Post-traumatic implant-supported restoration of the anterior maxillary teeth using cancellous bone block allografts. Journal of Oral and Maxillofacial Surgery. 2011;**69**(12):e513-e518

[44] Yamano S, Nissenbaum M, Dodson TB, Gallucci GO, Sukotjo C. Multidisciplinary treatment for a young patient with severe maxillofacial trauma from a snowmobile accident: A case report. The Journal of Oral Implantology. 2010;**36**(2):141-144

[45] Torabi K, Ahangari AH, Vojdani M, Fattahi F. Prosthodontic rehabilitation of a shotgun injury: A patient report. Journal of Prosthodontics. 2010;**19**(8):634-638

[46] Bidra AS, Veeranki AN. Surgical and prosthodontic reconstruction of a gunshot injury of the mandible using dental implants and an acrylic resin fixed prosthesis: A clinical report. The Journal of Prosthetic Dentistry. 2010;**104**(3):142-148

[47] Gökçen-Röhlig B, Atalay B, Baca E, Işik D, Meriç U. Prosthetic rehabilitation of a patient with a mandibular defect caused by a gunshot wound. The Journal of Craniofacial Surgery. 2009;**20**(5):1614-1617

[48] Sándor GKB, Carmichael RP. Rehabilitation of Trauma Using

Dental Implants. Atlas of the Oral and Maxillofacial Surgery Clinics. 2008;**16**(1):83-105

[49] Kao S-Y, Fong JH-J, Chou S-J, Wu J-H, Tu H-F, Yeung T-C. Segmental osteotomy to reposition multiple osseointegrated dental implants in the anterior maxilla in a trauma patient. Dental Traumatology. 2007;**23**(1):56-59

[50] Sipahi C, Ortakoglu K, Ozen J, Caglar A. The prosthodontic restoration of a self-inflicted gunshot maxillofacial defect: A short-term follow-up case report. The International Journal of Prosthodontics. 2007;**20**(1):85-88

[51] Cakan U, Anil N, Aslan Y. Prosthetic rehabilitation of a mandibular gunshot defect with an implant-supported fixed partial denture: A clinical report. The Journal of Prosthetic Dentistry. 2006;**95**(4):274-279

[52] Andersson L, Emami-Kristiansen Z, Högström J. Single-tooth implant treatment in the anterior region of the maxilla for treatment of tooth loss after trauma: A retrospective clinical and interview study. Dental Traumatology. 2003;**19**(3):126-131

[53] Tipton PA. Esthetic restoration of the traumatized and surgically reconstructed anterior maxilla. Journal of Esthetic and Restorative Dentistry. 2002;**14**(5):267-274

[54] De Angelis F, Papi P, Mencio F, Rosella D, Di Carlo S, Pompa G. Implant survival and success rates in patients with risk factors: Results from a long-term retrospective study with a 10 to 18 years follow-up. European Review for Medical and Pharmacological Sciences. 2017;**21**(3):433-437

[55] Radzewski R, Osmola K. The use of dental implants in organ transplant patients undergoing immunosuppressive therapy. Implant Dentistry. 2016;**25**(4):541-546

[56] Esfahanizadeh N, Yousefi H. Successful implant placement in a case of florid cemento-osseous dysplasia: A case report and literature review. The Journal of Oral Implantology. 2018;**44**(4):275-279

[57] Petrocelli M, Kretschmer W. Conservative treatment and implant rehabilitation of the mandible in a case of craniofacial fibrous dysplasia: A case report. Journal of Oral and Maxillofacial Surgery. 2014;**72**(5):902.e1-902.e6

[58] Bajwa MS, Ethunandan M, Flood TR. Oral rehabilitation with endosseous implants in a patient with fibrous dysplasia (McCune-Albright Syndrome): A case report. Journal of Oral and Maxillofacial Surgery. 2008;**66**(12):2605-2608

[59] de-Freitas N-R, Lima L-B, de-Moura M-B, Veloso-Guedes C-C-F, Simamoto-Júnior P-C, de-Magalhães D. Bisphosphonate treatment and dental implants: A systematic review. Medicina Oral, Patología Oral y Cirugía Bucal. 2016;**21**(5):e644-e651

[60] Ata-Ali J, Ata-Ali F, Peñarrocha-Oltra D, Galindo-Moreno P. What is the impact of bisphosphonate therapy upon dental implant survival? A systematic review and meta-analysis. Clinical Oral Implants Research. 2016;**27**(2):e38-e46

[61] Ferlito S, Liardo C, Puzzo S. Bisphosponates and dental implants: A case report and a brief review of literature. Minerva Stomatologica. 2011;**60**(1-2):75-81

[62] Bedogni A, Bettini G, Totola A, Saia G, Nocini PF. Oral bisphosphonate-associated osteonecrosis of the jaw after implant surgery: A case report and literature review. Journal of Oral and Maxillofacial Surgery. 2010;**68**(7):1662-1666

[63] Javed F, Almas K. Osseointegration of dental implants in patients

undergoing bisphosphonate treatment: A literature review. Journal of Periodontology. 2010;**81**(4):479-484

[64] Madrid C, Sanz M. What impact do systemically administrated bisphosphonates have on oral implant therapy? A systematic review. Clinical Oral Implants Research. 2009;**20**(4):87-95

[65] Javed F, Romanos GE. Impact of diabetes mellitus and glycemic control on the osseointegration of dental implants: A systematic literature review. Journal of Periodontology. 2009;**80**(11):1719-1730

[66] Ormianer Z, Block J, Matalon S, Kohen J. The effect of moderately controlled type 2 diabetes on dental implant survival and peri-implant bone loss: A long-term retrospective study. The International Journal of Oral & Maxillofacial Implants. 2018;**33**(2):389-394

[67] de Araújo Nobre M, Maló P, Gonçalves Y, Sabas A, Salvado F. Dental implants in diabetic patients: Retrospective cohort study reporting on implant survival and risk indicators for excessive marginal bone loss at 5 years. Journal of Oral Rehabilitation. 2016;**43**(11):863-870

[68] Nobre M de A, Maló P, Gonçalves Y, Sabas A, Salvado F. Outcome of dental implants in diabetic patients with and without cardiovascular disease: A 5-year post-loading retrospective study. European Journal of Oral Implantology. 2016;**9**(1):87-95

[69] Hurst D. Evidence unclear on whether Type I or II diabetes increases the risk of implant failure. Evidence-Based Dentistry. 2014;**15**(4):102-103

[70] Hwang D, Wang H-L. Medical contraindications to implant therapy: Part I: Absolute contraindications. Implant Dentistry. 2006;**15**(4):353-360

[71] Doğan GE, Halici Z, Karakus E, Erdemci B, Alsaran A, Cinar I. Dose-dependent effect of radiation on resorbable blast material titanium implants: An experimental study in rabbits. Acta Odontologica Scandinavica. 2018;**76**(2):130-134

[72] Nack C, Raguse J-D, Stricker A, Nelson K, Nahles S. Rehabilitation of irradiated patients with chemically modified and conventional SLA implants: Five-year follow-up. Journal of Oral Rehabilitation. 2015;**42**(1):57-64

[73] Chambrone L, Mandia J, Shibli JA, Romito GA, Abrahao M. Dental implants installed in irradiated jaws. Journal of Dental Research. 2013;**92**(12_suppl):119S-130S

[74] Esposito M, Worthington HV. Interventions for replacing missing teeth: Hyperbaric oxygen therapy for irradiated patients who require dental implants. Cochrane Database of Systematic Reviews. 2013;**30**(9):CD003603

[75] Ella B, Lasserre J-F, Blanchard J-P, Fricain JC. A 4-year follow-up of two complete mandibular implant-supported removable prostheses in a patient with severe rheumatoid polyarthritis: Case report. The International Journal of Oral & Maxillofacial Implants. 2011;**26**(2):e19-e22

[76] Krennmair G, Seemann R, Piehslinger E. Dental implants in patients with rheumatoid arthritis: Clinical outcome and peri-implant findings. Journal of Clinical Periodontology. 2010;**37**(10):928-936

[77] Weinlander M, Krennmair G, Piehslinger E. Implant prosthodontic rehabilitation of patients with rheumatic disorders: A case series report. The International Journal of Prosthodontics. 2010;**23**(1):22-28

[78] Almeida D, Vianna K, Arriaga P, Moraschini V. Dental implants in Sjögren's syndrome patients: A systematic review. PLoS One. 2017;**12**(12):e0189507

[79] Ergun S, Katz J, Cifter ED, Koray M, Esen BA, Tanyeri H. Implant-supported oral rehabilitation of a patient with systemic lupus erythematosus: Case report and review of the literature. Quintessence International. 2010;**41**(10):863-867

[80] Kinaia BM, Hope K, Zuhaili A, Tulasne JF. Full-mouth rehabilitation with calvarium bone grafts and dental implants for a papillon-lefèvre syndrome patient: Case report. The International Journal of Oral & Maxillofacial Implants. 2017;**32**(6):e259-e264

[81] Al Farraj AlDosari A. Oral rehabilitation of a case of Papillon-Lefevre syndrome with dental implants. Saudi Medical Journal. 2013;**34**(4):424-427

[82] Senel FC et al. A 3-year follow-up of the rehabilitation of Papillon-Lefèvre syndrome by dental implants. Journal of Oral and Maxillofacial Surgery. 2012;**70**(1):163-167

[83] Kramer F-J, Baethge C, Tschernitschek H. Implants in children with ectodermal dysplasia: A case report and literature review. Clinical Oral Implants Research. 2007;**18**(1):140-146

[84] Kutkut A, Abu-Eid R, Sharab L, Abadi B, Van Sickels J. Full mouth implant-supported rehabilitation of a patient with ectodermal dysplasia: Clinical report and literature review. Journal of the International Academy of Periodontology. 2015;**17**(2):34-41

[85] Wang Y, He J, Decker AM, Hu JC, Zou D. Clinical outcomes of implant therapy in ectodermal dysplasia patients: A systematic review. International Journal of Oral and Maxillofacial Surgery. 2016;**45**(8):1035-1043

[86] Bergendal B, Bjerklin K, Bergendal T, Koch G. Dental implant therapy for a child with X-linked hypohidrotic ectodermal dysplasia—Three decades of managed care. The International Journal of Prosthodontics. 2015;**28**(4):348-356

[87] Clauss F, Waltmann E, Barriere P, Hadj-Rabia S, Manière M-C, Schmittbuhl M. Dento-maxillo-facial phenotype and implants-based oral rehabilitation in Ectodermal Dysplasia with WNT10A gene mutation: Report of a case and literature review. Journal of Cranio-Maxillofacial Surgery. 2014;**42**(6):e346-e351

[88] Baptist BA. Fixed implant supported rehabilitation of partially edentulous posterior maxilla in a patient with systemic scleroderma. Implant Dentistry. 2016;**25**(1):155-159

[89] Zigdon H, Gutmacher Z, Teich S, Levin L. Full-mouth rehabilitation using dental implants in a patient with scleroderma. Quintessence International. 2011;**42**(9):781-785

[90] Nam J, Janakievski J, Raigrodski AJ. Complete transition from failing restorations to implant-supported fixed prostheses in a patient with scleroderma. The Compendium of Continuing Education in Dentistry. 2012;**33**(10):746-756

[91] Gómez-de Diego R, Mang-de la Rosa M del R, Romero-Pérez M-J, Cutando-Soriano A, López-Valverde-Centeno A. Indications and contraindications of dental implants in medically compromised patients: Update. Medicina Oral, Patología Oral y Cirugía Bucal. 2014;**19**(5):e483-e489

[92] Odman J, Gröndahl K, Lekholm U, Thilander B. The effect of osseointegrated implants on the

dento-alveolar development. A clinical and radiographic study in growing pigs. European Journal of Orthodontics. 1991;**13**(4):279-286

[93] Thilander B, Odman J, Gröndahl K, Lekholm U. Aspects on osseointegrated implants inserted in growing jaws. A biometric and radiographic study in the young pig. European Journal of Orthodontics. 1992;**14**(2):99-109

[94] Sennerby L, Odman J, Lekholm U, Thilander B. Tissue reactions towards titanium implants inserted in growing jaws. A histological study in the pig. Clinical Oral Implants Research. 1993;**4**(2):65-75

[95] Smalley WM, Shapiro PA, Hohl TH, Kokich VG, Brånemark PI. Osseointegrated titanium implants for maxillofacial protraction in monkeys. American Journal of Orthodontics and Dentofacial Orthopedics. 1988;**94**(4):285-295

[96] Cronin RJ, Oesterle LJ. Implant use in growing patients. Treatment planning concerns. Dental Clinics of North America. 1998;**42**(1):1-34

[97] Bjork A. Variations in the growth pattern of the human mandible: Longitudinal radiographic study by the implant method. Journal of Dental Research. 1963;**42**(1 Pt 2):400-411

[98] Thilander B, Odman J, Gröndahl K, Friberg B. Osseointegrated implants in adolescents. An alternative in replacing missing teeth? European Journal of Orthodontics. 1994;**16**(2):84-95

[99] Roberts WE, Helm FR, Marshall KJ, Gongloff RK. Rigid endosseous implants for orthodontic and orthopedic anchorage. The Angle Orthodontist. 1989;**59**(4):247-256

[100] Oesterle LJ, Cronin RJ, Ranly DM. Maxillary implants and the growing patient. The International Journal of Oral & Maxillofacial Implants. 1993;**8**(4):377-387

[101] Cronin RJ, Oesterle LJ, Ranly DM. Mandibular implants and the growing patient. The International Journal of Oral & Maxillofacial Implants. 1994;**9**(1):55-62

[102] Maiorana C, Speroni S, Herford AS, Cicciù M. Slow orthodontic teeth extrusion to enhance hard and soft periodontal tissue quality before implant positioning in aesthetic area. The Open Dentistry Journal. 2012;**6**(1):137-142

[103] Adell R, Lekholm U, Rockler B, Brånemark PI. A 15-year study of osseointegrated implants in the treatment of the edentulous jaw. International Journal of Oral Surgery. 1981;**10**(6):387-416

[104] Kleinheinz J, Büchter A, Kruse-Lösler B, Weingart D, Joos U. Incision design in implant dentistry based on vascularization of the mucosa. Clinical Oral Implants Research. 2005;**16**(5):518-523

[105] Cameron HU, Pilliar RM, MacNab I. The effect of movement on the bonding of porous metal to bone. Journal of Biomedical Materials Research. 1973;7(4):301-311

[106] Szmukler-Moncler S, Piattelli A, Favero GA, Dubruille JH. Considerations preliminary to the application of early and immediate loading protocols in dental implantology. Clinical Oral Implants Research. 2000;**11**(1):12-25

[107] Kawahara H, Kawahara D, Hayakawa M, Tamai Y, Kuremoto T, Matsuda S. Osseointegration under immediate loading: Biomechanical stress-strain and bone formation—Resorption. Implant Dentistry. 2003;**12**(1):61-68

[108] Meyer U et al. Ultrastructural characterization of the implant/ bone interface of immediately loaded dental implants. Biomaterials. 2004;**25**(10):1959-1967

[109] Misch CE, Wang H-L, Misch CM, Sharawy M, Lemons J, Judy KWM. Rationale for the application of immediate load in implant dentistry: Part I. Implant Dentistry. 2004;**13**(3):207-217

[110] Meyer U, Wiesmann H-P, Fillies T, Joos U. Early tissue reaction at the interface of immediately loaded dental implants. The International Journal of Oral & Maxillofacial Implants. 2003;**18**(4):489-499

[111] Nkenke E et al. Bone contact, growth, and density around immediately loaded implants in the mandible of mini pigs. Clinical Oral Implants Research. 2003;**14**(3):312-321

[112] Açil Y, Sievers J, Gülses A, Ayna M, Wiltfang J, Terheyden H. Correlation between resonance frequency, insertion torque and bone-implant contact in self-cutting threaded implants. Odontology. 2017;**105**(3):347-353

[113] Trisi P, Berardini M, Falco A, Podaliri Vulpiani M. Validation of value of actual micromotion as a direct measure of implant micromobility after healing (secondary implant stability). An *in vivo* histologic and biomechanical study. Clinical Oral Implants Research. 2016;**27**(11):1423-1430

[114] Levin BP. The correlation between immediate implant insertion torque and implant stability quotient. The International Journal of Periodontics & Restorative Dentistry. 2016;**36**(6):833-840

[115] Khoury J, Ghosn N, Mokbel N, Naaman N. Buccal bone thickness overlying maxillary anterior teeth. Implant Dentistry. 2016;**25**(4):525-531

[116] Zhang W, Skrypczak A, Weltman R. Anterior maxilla alveolar ridge dimension and morphology measurement by cone beam computerized tomography (CBCT) for immediate implant treatment planning. BMC Oral Health. 2015;**15**(1):65

[117] Vera C et al. Evaluation of buccal alveolar bone dimension of maxillary anterior and premolar teeth: A cone beam computed tomography investigation. The International Journal of Oral & Maxillofacial Implants;**27**(6):1514-1519

[118] Saffarpour A et al. Bactericidal effect of erbium-doped yttrium aluminum garnet laser and photodynamic therapy on aggregatibacter actinomycetemcomitans biofilm on implant surface. The International Journal of Oral & Maxillofacial Implants. 2016;**31**(3):e71-e78

[119] Natto ZS, Aladmawy M, Levi PA, Wang H-L. Comparison of the efficacy of different types of lasers for the treatment of peri-implantitis: A systematic review. The International Journal of Oral & Maxillofacial Implants. 2015;**30**(2):338-345

[120] Kreisler M et al. Bactericidal effect of the Er:YAG laser on dental implant surfaces: An in vitro study. Journal of Periodontology. 2002;**73**(11):1292-1298

Section 3

Material

Chapter 3

Biomaterial Used in Trauma Patients

Mehmet Yaltirik, Meltem Koray, Hümeyra Kocaelli, Duygu Ofluoglu and Cevat Tugrul Turgut

Abstract

The development of bone tissue engineering and bone regeneration is always of interest to improve methods to reduce costs of trauma patient. Ability to use autogenous bone forming cells attached to bone morphogenetic proteins would be ideal. There are many clinical reasons to develop bone tissue engineering alternatives, for use in the reconstruction of large defects and implants. The traditional methods of bone defect management include autografting and allografting cancellous bone, vascularized grafts, and other bone transport techniques. However, these are the standard treatments. Since bone grafts are avascular and dependent on the size of the defect, the viability can limit their application. In large defects, the grafts can be resorbed by the body before osteogenesis is complete; tissue loss develops in the living organism due to infection, trauma, congenital, and physiological reasons. Placing tissue defects in the dentist and maxillofacial surgery and accelerating wound healing are an important issue. From an old Egypt, material used in treatment of different doctors with various causes. Oral surgery, periodontology, and implantology, which are surgical branches of the dentistry, need to increase bone formation in the treatment of bone defects, congenital defects, and defects around the implant. Many years of work have been done to obtain ideal biomaterials, and many materials have been used. We have prepared detailed information on biomaterials used in dentistry, oral, and maxillofacial surgeries in this book to help dentists and dental students.

Keywords: biomaterials, trauma, maxillofacial surgery

1. Introduction

Bone not only supports and protects various organs but it also facilitates mobility [1], with the help of the soft collagen protein and stiffer apatite mineral. Bone is maintained dynamically through two different processes: modeling and remodeling [2]. In bone modeling process, the new bone is formed without prior bone resorption, while in the bone remodeling process, bone formation follows bone resorption [1]. Bone remodeling is a lifelong process that begins in early fetal life and is maintaining bone function by continuously replacing damaged bone with new bone tissue [3, 4].

The use of alloplastic materials in the remodelization of traumatized lesions and fractures in the compensation of tissues lost for various reasons such as trauma first started in ancient Egypt [5]. All substances are called biomaterials, which help to eliminate any deficiencies in the living organism and help the organism to complete this deficiency regularly and quickly [5].

Bone grafting is one of the most common surgical procedures to set up bone regeneration procedures [6]. Bone grafting procedures were the second most frequent tissue transplantation after blood transfusion [7]. Autologous bone is still gold standard in bone regeneration [8]. Bone grafting procedures vary between natural grafts to synthetic bone substitutes and biological factors [9]. Synthetic bone substitutes and biological factors, calcium phosphate (CaP)-based biomaterials (e.g., hydroxyapatite (HAp), CaP cements, and ceramics), and recombinant human bone morphological proteins (rhBMPs) are most frequently used [10].

This chapter will describe the biomaterials used in the reconstruction of defects in the head and neck region [5].

2. Structure of bone

Bone is a connective tissue that forms the skeleton of the body, acts as a support to the muscles and organs, protects them against. Bone tissue consists of two different bone structures as compact or cortical spongiosa or cancellous bone [5].

Bone tissue is examined in two separate parts: the matrix between the cells and the cells [5].

2.1 Cells

2.1.1 Osteoprogenitor cells

These cells are the result of differentiation of stromal cells arising from embryonal mesenchymal cells in periosteum and endosteum. Cells related to direct bone formation are osteoblasts, osteocytes, connective tissue, fibroblast, and fat cells.

2.1.2 Osteoblasts

They play a role in the synthesis, preparation, and mineralization of the bone matrix. They are then implanted into the tissue with calcification of the bone matrix to become osteocytes.

2.1.3 Osteocytes

They surround with osteoblasts, mineral matrix and then consequent balance of the calcium (Ca) level.

2.1.4 Bone marrow cells

They are cells similar to squamous epithelial cells found in inactive regions in the bone.

2.1.5 Osteoclasts

Osteoclasts digest the mineral matrix of the bone with acid phosphatase, which they secrete, and then resorb it by digesting collagen and other organic matrix structures with lysosomal enzymes.

2.2 The intercellular tissue (bone matrix)

Cell-to-cell tissue forms 10–29% water, 60–70% of the bone dry weight is the inorganic structure (bone salts), and 30–40% of the bone dry weight, 90–96% of the organic structure is collagen, which is also the main component of connective tissue and constitutes one-third of all body proteins [5].

3. Healing mechanism of bone defects

Bone repair can be defined in two procedures: primary bone healing and secondary bone healing. The large segmental bone loss in the defect is an extreme condition in bone healing, which can be caused by trauma, diseases, developmental deformities, revision surgery, and tumor resection or osteomyelitis [11, 12].

Primary (direct) bone healing mainly happens when the fracture gap is less than 0.1 mm, and the fracture site is rigidly stabilized. Secondary bone healing is the more common form of bone healing and occurs when the fracture edges are less than twice the diameter of the injured bone [11]. Blood clothing, inflammatory response, fibrocartilage callus formation, membranous ossifications, and bone modeling are involved in bone healing.

Bone substitutes mainly involve three important biological properties: osteogenesis osteoinduction, and osteoconduction [13].

3.1 Bone formation mechanism with bone graft materials

3.1.1 Osteogenesis

Bone graft materials in osteogenesis include organic materials that have bone formation capacity directly from osteoblast cells. Even in environments where undifferentiated mesenchymal cells are not present in the tissue, such organic materials have the ability to be osteogenic. The only graft material with osteogenic character is autogenous bone. Autogenous bone is obtained from the oral surgery, iliac bone, tuber maxilla, and mandibular symphysis [5].

3.1.2 Osteoinduction

Osteoinduction, with osteoinductive materials, has the capacity to convert undifferentiated mesenchymal cells in tissue into osteoblasts and chondroblasts. In oral surgery, bone allografts are the most commonly used osteoinductive materials. Bone allograft is derived from different human bone tissues with different genetic structure.

3.1.3 Osteoconduction

The growth of bone tissue with osteoconduction is characterized by the formation of appositional bone. That is why osteoconduction occurs in the presence of bone or undifferentiated mesenchymal cells.

As a result, although bone has a very variable metabolism, resistance depends on the amount of collagen, the arrangement of fibrils, the presence of minerals, and the presence of minerals on proteins and glucosamines.

4. Basic features of biomaterials

1. Biological suitability: the applied biomaterial should be acceptable to the tissue [5].
2. It should be bioinert and biocompatible. It should be osteoconductive and osteogenic.
3. The surface should have an immediate stabilization property and surface porosity to allow for increased stabilization.
4. It should not be toxic.
5. It must be easily sterilized.
6. It must be resistant to infection.
7. There should be no color features that can affect surrounding textures.
8. It must be easy to apply and must cause minimal trauma during application.
9. It must be resistant to bending and twisting and should be elastic; elasticity should be close to the applied texture. It must be cut and shaped during application.
10. Resorption should be resistant.
11. The application must be acceptable to the patient.
12. The application should be able to give definite results.
13. It is easy to remove or cut in case of failure.
14. Must be easy to store.
15. It must be cheap and easy to obtain.

5. Classification of biomaterials

A. Bone source biomaterials [5]

a. Autogenous bone graft (autograft)

I. Cortical and cancellous bone in or out of mouth

b. Homogeneous bone graft (allograft)

I. Isograft: fresh cancellous bone marrow

II. Fresh frozen bone

III. Frozen dried bone

c. Heterogeneous bone graft (xenograft)

I. Demineralized bone

II. Protein-extracted bone

B. Bone-free biomaterials (alloplastics)

a. Tissue sources

I. Dentin

II. Cementum

III. Cartilage

IV. Sclera

V. Dura mater, etc.

b. Metals

c. Gelatin film

d. Polymers

e. Calcium sulfate

f. Calcium carbonate

g. Calcium phosphates

h. Calcium phosphate ceramics (CaP ceramics)

i. Bioactive glass

5.1 Bone source biomaterials

In the treatment of traumatic defects, congenital deformities, tumor surgery are in used. Today, homogeneous bone grafts (allografts), heterogeneous bone grafts (xenografts), and alloplastic materials are used in oral and maxillofacial surgery [5].

An osseous graft from an anatomic site and transplanted to another site within the same individuals is called autologous bone grafting [14, 15]. With osteoconductive, osteoinductive, and osteogenic properties, an autologous bone graft can integrate into the host bone more rapidly and completely [15]; therefore, it is regarded as the gold standard bone defects [16].

Cancellous autografts are the most commonly used form. Few osteoblasts and osteocytes, but abundant mesenchymal stem cells (MSCs), survive as a result of ischemia during transplantation, which helps maintaining osteogenic potential and the ability to generate new bone from the graft [17]. Autograft-derived proteins, which are attributed to the osteoinduction of the graft, are also preserved and present when the autografts are appropriately treated [15, 18].

Cortical autografts have excellent structure and are mechanically supportive, due to osteoprogenitor cells [14]. Unlike the autologous cancellous graft, the creeping substitution of cortical autograft is mainly mediated by osteoclasts after the rapid hematoma formation and inflammatory response in early phase of bone regeneration, since the revascularization and remodeling processes are strictly hampered by the dense architecture [15].

5.1.1 Autogenous bone graft (autograft)

Autogenous grafts: the fresh autogenous graft taken from the same organism contains osteogenic cells and does not cause an immunological reaction; this group is the most advantageous graft material. However, the disadvantages of this group include the need for a second operation in the donor area, long-term postoperative pain and limitation of movement, and prolonged maintenance. Autogenous bone grafts can be obtained from crista iliaca: grafts costal grafts and cranial bones, structurally separated as cortical bone, cancellous, and corticocancellous bone [5].

Intraoral cancellous bone: Upper jaw tuber region, toothless regions, exocytoses, recovery sites ramus mandibula, interlobar alveolar bone, lower jaw semispherical region and ramus mandibula, and bone fragments arising during operation [5].

Oral cancellous bone: The iliac bone is obtained from bone, ribs, and other endochondral bones.

Corticocancellous bone: The corticocancellous bone does not have the osteogenesis-enhancing properties as cancellous bone. This type of graft is most commonly of rib or ilium origin [5].

5.1.2 Homogeneous bone graft (homograft)

An autogenous bone graft is obtained from the individual itself.

Isograft: The tissues taken from living things with the same genetic structure as the recipient are called isografts or syngenesioplastic grafts.

Allografts are tissues from the same species but from living things that are genetically identical to the recipient. Bone allografts are obtained from human beings of different genetic types and from bones extracted from humans, such as cadavers or hip fractures, and are maintained in bone banks by a series of procedures [11]. It has many advantages compared to being obtained from living people. The advantages are elimination of donor site, reduction of anesthesia and duration of operation, loss of blood loss and complications at low level. The disadvantage is that the touch is taken by another person [5].

Considering the limitation of autologous bone grafts is the best alternative to autografts and has been used effectively in clinical practice in many cases, especially for patients who have poor healing potential, established nonunion, and extensive comminution after fractures [15, 17]. The allograft may be machined and customized and is therefore available in a variety of forms, including cortical, cancellous, and highly processed bone derivatives [14]. Allografts are found to be immunogenic and have higher failure rate, which are believed to be caused by activation of major histocompatibility complex [19].

Cancellous allografts are the most common types of commercial allogeneic grafts and are supplied predominately in the form of blocks [14]. Compared to autografts, a similar but slower sequence of events happens in the incorporation process of allografts [15].

Cortical allografts confer rigid mechanical properties and are mainly applied in spinal augmentation for filling large defects [14]. In consideration of immune responses and for safety, frozen or freeze dried products that are free of marrow and blood are commonly transplanted [15].

Demineralized bone matrix is highly processed allograft derivative with at least 40% of the mineral content of the bone matrix removed by the acid, while collagens, noncollagenous proteins, and growth factors remain [17].

Demineralized bone matrix osteoconductivity is conferred by providing a framework for cell populating and for generating new bone after the treatment [18]. Osteoinductive property of demineralized bone matrix is mainly determined by the remaining growth factors, which are directly correlated with preparation methods. Demineralized bone matrix is similar to that of the autogenous graft, with growth factors triggering an endochondral ossification cascade and culminating in new bone formation at the site of implantation [18].

Recent techniques in preparing immunoglobulin complications of allografts to remove the disease carrying potentials are freezing, freezing and drying, or exposure to radiation. The applied bone has a slower revascularization and more resorptive activity than autogenous grafts [5].

The mechanism of revascularization begins with an acute infinite response and lasts for a long time, followed by chronic infilamations. It meets cellular immunological response in frozen bone applications.

5.1.3 Heterogeneous bone graft (xenograft)

Heterogeneous bone grafts are called grafts from a different species. The heterogeneous term is used for tissues from different species. Heterogeneous bone grafts have been proposed to fill small jaw defects, and many clinicians have indicated that these grafts have any osteogenic potential but instead are matrix for bone formation. Studies done with inorganic calf bone showed successful results in graft osteotomy sites but not in posttraumatic deformity and hypoplastic area corrections [5].

5.1.3.1 Clinical use of the allogeneic bone

Allogeneic bones prepared for different frozen, dried, or frozen oral surgical procedures are available in different anatomical shapes. Cancerous iliac bone is divided into particles of about 2–10 mm in diameter for use in bone defects. Small cancellous particles are used in the periapical areas after curettage with limited alveolar edge corrections [5].

Researchers who have expected to make use of osteoconductive effects of alloplastic bone materials (hydroxylapatite, tricalcium phosphate, etc.) and bone allografts and autogenous bone grafts cause postoperative complications in the donor area have been directed to obtain bone grafts with both osseoinductive and osseoconductive allogenic, low antigenic properties. For this purpose, autolyzed, degenerated (allogenic) bone was studied. In contrast to lyophilized or other allogenic human bones, researchers indicate that the allogenic bone is osteoconductive. The use of lyophilized and sterile human allogenic bone in parts or powder forms is offered. The powder forms of this bone are suggested for filling the cyst cavity [5].

5.2 Bone-free biomaterials (alloplasts)

Allogenic grafts which lost vitality have been seen, organic, and inorganic inanimate materials and synthetic materials obtained from animals such as ceramic hydroxylapatites, tricalcium phosphates, and various "alloplastic materials."

The most important problem in the alloplastic material is the tendency of the immunological system to encapsulate and isolate foreign bodies [5].

Alloplasts have been using in bone defects due to various reasons, such as cranial, mandibular, maxillary, nasal, zygomatic, TME reconstructions, or traumatic augmentations, are metals, polymers, hydroxylapatite, and associated calcium triphosphate ceramics or combinations of these materials.

5.2.1 Tissue sources

I. Dentin: It consists of hydroxyapatite crystals with a strong structure. This crystal structure is histologically resistant and resistant to osteoblast, osteoclast, blood vessel, and nerve tissue in a strong collagen network.

II. Cement: It is a bony matter that is directly related to the collagen fibers of the jawbone through the periodontal membrane.

III. Cartilage

IV. Sclera

V. Dura mater

5.2.2 Metals

Metal biomaterials are widely used in electrosurgical surgery, orthognathic surgery, and orthopedic surgery. Metallic stiffness is a desirable feature for implants that will encounter load force, especially during functioning. The metal groups used are alloys such as gold, platinum, stainless steel, titanium, and chromium-cobalt.

Bioinorganic ions, such as silicon, magnesium, strontium, zinc, and copper, can still be regarded as essential cofactors of enzymes, coenzymes, or prosthetic groups [20].

Mechanism of magnesium ions on fracture healing is not yet fully explained; recent investigations showed that the osteogenerative effect of Mg^{2+} on undifferentiated human bone marrow stromal cells (hBMSCs) and osteogenic hBMSCs was likely attributed to connected the subsequent orchestrated [20].

Strontium to reduce bone resorption and osteoclast activity [20] were also observed under rat osteoclasts and primary mature rabbit osteoclasts, respectively. The adverse effect of strontium in cardiovascular diseases and venous thrombosis has been highlighted [20].

Silicon is a silica-based synthetic bone substitute, which is used in orthopedic; bioglass cannot be ignored when discussing the effect of silicon on bone regeneration. Bioglass has a key role because of the fact that the hydroxyapatite coating, but not the leaching silicon ions, played an active role in the processes leading to new bone formation [19]. Zinc is involved in the structural, catalytic, or regulatory action of several important metalloenzymes, and alkaline phosphatase (ALP) is among them. ALP not only generates phosphates by hydrolyzing pyrophosphates but also creates an alkaline environment, which favored the precipitation and subsequent mineralization of these phosphates in the extracellular matrix, which were produced by osteoblasts [20].

Copper has been recognized as a cofactor for several other enzymes in body, one of which is related to the musculoskeletal system [20]. Lithium has attracted attention due to its role in osteogenesis [20]. Like copper, cobalt was recently showed to stimulate angiogenesis [20].

5.2.3 Gelatin film

It can be used as resurfacing, porous, nonantigenic, and in the middle ear surgery for pleural injuries in dura mater application.

5.2.4 Polymers

Polymethylmethacrylates are self-polymerized acrylics that are identified as bone cement.

Polymethylmethacrylate (PMMA) remains a key component of modern practice and is nonbiodegradable and nonresorbable, which makes it more like grouting than cement, and thus cannot be considered a bone substitute material, which is used in clinics [19].

5.2.5 Calcium sulfate

When combined with other synthetic bone substitutes and/or growth factors [20], one of the promising approaches is to load antibiotics to this biomaterial.

5.2.6 Calcium carbonate

The outer layer of corals in the calcium carbonate structure releases a calcareous substance called aragonite. The physical structure is similar to cancellous bone and consists of trace elements such as 98% calcium carbonate, 2% fluorine, zinc, copper, iron, and strontium. It is an excellent tissue-compatible material that can completely resurface during the healing process and has an osteoconductive effect on new bone formation [5].

5.2.7 Calcium phosphate

Calcium phosphate material is similar to HA in terms of its behavior in the tissue. However, calcium phosphate has the most pronounced multiplication property, which is closely related to bone without the need for porosity.

5.2.8 Calcium phosphate ceramics (CaP ceramics)

Calcium phosphate ceramics are calcium hydroxyapatites, which is a chemical composition similar to the mineral phase of calcified tissues [17]. Hydroxyapatite (HAp) is occurring mineral form of calcium apatite with the formula of $Ca_{10}[PO_4]6[OH]_2$ and comprises about 50% of the weight of the bone, which accounts for its excellent osteoconductive and osteointegrative properties [14, 17].

5.2.9 Bioactive glass

Bioactive glass, known as bioglass, refers to a synthetic silicate-based ceramics and was originally constituted by silicon dioxide (SiO_2), sodium oxide (Na_2O), calcium oxide (CaO), and phosphorus pentoxide (P_2O_5) [20]. The optimized constitutions lead to a strong physical bonding between bioglass and host bone. If hydroxyapatite coating on the surface of bioglass takes place, it absorbs proteins and attracts osteoprogenitor cells [20].

6. Principles of biomaterial trauma applications

Correcting the deformities, the first thing to note in augmentation is the presence of the epithelium that can cover the implanted material completely and without tension. In cases where deformity is common and tissue loss is large, skin and soft tissue transplantation may be required before biomaterial is applied. If the defect in the bone tissue is too large, graft should be considered, and functional stress in the receiving area, load, and the trauma to it should be considered.

Bone defect may result in delayed union or even nonunion if the treatment is improper. Therefore, bone grafting techniques should take place in the surgical process. Even though various synthetic bone substitutes offer diversity options, the treatment outcome is still incomparable to the autologous bone graft in terms of bone healing quality and time management. Ions such as magnesium, strontium, silicon, copper, and cobalt are feasible solution for bone defect. Therapeutic effect and mechanism of ions have been understood. Bioinorganic ions can be applied with growth factors and induce new bone formation.

Every surgeon should use the technique in the direction of the prepared plan, determine the biomaterial, and apply it on the model. Atraumatic work should be performed as much as possible during the operation, the material used should conform to the defect contours, the stabilization should be esthetic of the patient, and the appropriate tools should be used in the biomaterials during surgery to manipulate the material so as not to create sharp or irregular edges. Stabilization is provided by sewing, wire, and nails. Good closure of the incision is important in the postoperative period. Careful evaluation of each phase will ultimately bring success.

Acknowledgements

This chapter was performed by Mehmet Yaltirik, Meltem Koray, Hümeyra Kocaelli, Duygu Ofluoglu, and Cevat Tugrul Turgut in Istanbul University, Faculty of Dentistry, Department of Oral and Maxillofacial Surgery.

Conflict of interest

We declare that there is no conflict of interest with any financial organization regarding the material discussed in the chapter.

Author details

Mehmet Yaltirik*, Meltem Koray, Hümeyra Kocaelli, Duygu Ofluoglu and Cevat Tugrul Turgut
Department of Oral and Maxillofacial Surgery, Faculty of Dentistry, Istanbul University, Turkey

*Address all correspondence to: mehmet.yaltirik@istanbul.edu.tr

References

[1] Fonseca RJ, Walker RV. Oral and Maxillofacial Trauma. Vol. II. Philadelphia, WB: Saunders Company; 1991

[2] Guyton AC. Tibbi Fizyoloji. In: Textbook of Medical Physiology. 7th ed. Philadelphia: WB Saunder Company; 1986. pp. 937-953

[3] Kikırdak GY. Kemik ve Biyokimyasl. İ.Ü.Diş.Hek.Fak. Biyokimya Bilim Dali Ders NotIan. 1988:**37**;300-391

[4] Jaffe HL. Metabolic, Degenerative and Inflammatory Diseases of Bones and Joints. Munchen, Berlin, Wien: Urban and Schwarzenberg; 1972. pp. 44-104

[5] Tuskan C, Yaltirik M. Oral ve Mksillofasiyal Cerrahide Kullanılan Biyomateryaller. İstanbul: Istanbul Universitesi Yayinlari İstanbul; 2002. pp. 1-54

[6] Amler MH, LeGeros RZ. Hard tissue replacement polymer as an implant material. Journal of Biomedical Materials Research. 1992;**24**:1079-1089

[7] Archer WH. Oral and Maxillofacial Surgery. 5th ed. Vol. II, 1975. Philadelphia: WB Saunders Company. pp. 1512-1526

[8] Aukhil I, Simpson DM, Sugss C, Petterson E. In vivo differentiation of progeniton cells of the periodontal ligament. An experimental study using physical barriers. Journal of Clinical Periodontology. 1986;**13**:862-868

[9] Bovde A, Wolfe LA, Jones SJ, Vesely P, Maly M. Microscopy of bone cells, bone tissue and bone healing around implants. Implant Dentistry. 1992;**1**:117-125

[10] Braley S. The silicones in maxillofacial surgery. Laryngoscope. 1968;**78**:549

[11] Kasaboğlu Ç. Normal ve diabetli stçanlarda kemik travmasmdan sonra kan serumunda görülen degişiklilerin incelenmesi [thesis]. Istanbul: Istanbul Universitesi; 1986

[12] Nayir E. DişhekimIiği Maddeler Bilgisi. 7th ed. İstanbul; 1999. pp. 25-39

[13] Schaffer AB. The combined use of hydroxyapatite segments and granules for alveolar ridge reconstruction. Oral and Maxillofacial Surgery. 1993;**51**:26

[14] Smith EL, Hill RL, Lehman R, Lefkowitz R J, Handler F, White A, Principles of Bio-chemistry. International student ed. 1983. pp. 15-18

[15] Soydan N. Genel Histoloji, Taş Matbaası. Istanbul: Istanbul Universitesi; 1985. pp. 100-119

[16] Wismeijer D, Vermeeren JIJH, Van Waas MAJ. Patient satisfaction with overdentures supported by one-stage TPS implants. The International Journal of Oral & Maxillofacial Implants. 1992;**7**:51-55

[17] Albrektsonn T, Zarb G, Worthington P, Ericsson A. The long term efficacy of currently used dental implants. Journal of Oral and Maxillofacial Implants. 1986;**1**:11-25

[18] Sandalll F, Karabuda C. Oral implantolojide kemik grefti materyalleri ve kullamlan. Oral Implantoloji Dergisi. 1999;**1**:9-16

[19] Bouchard P, Ouhayoun JP, Nilveus RE. Expanded polytetrafluoroethylene membranes and connective tissue grafts support bone regeneration for closing mandibular Class II furcations. Journal of Clinical Periodontology. 1993;**54**:1193-1198

[20] Wang W, Yeung KWK. Bone grafts and biomaterials substitutes for bone defect repair: A review. Bioactive Materials. 2017;**2**:224-247

Section 4

Pediatrics

Chapter 4

Dental Traumatology in Pediatric Dentistry

Asli Topaloglu Ak, Didem Oner Ozdas, Sevgi Zorlu and Pinar Kiymet Karataban

Abstract

In this chapter, epidemiology of dental trauma will be discussed in terms of its incidence and prevalence among primary and permanent dentition. Dental trauma causes and its distribution in accordance with age and sex will be highlighted. Classification of dental trauma based on soft and hard tissue injuries will be outlined, and subsequently, clinical examination and diagnosis will be featured. Treatment modalities and variations between permanent and primary dentition will be discussed along with the new treatment era namely regenerative approach and decoronation. Splints, techniques, and follow-up routines will also be discussed. Last but not least, prevention of dental trauma will be discussed.

Keywords: dental trauma, children, splints, classification

1. An epidemiological approach to dental traumatology

Traumatic dental injuries are a public dental health problem worldwide and can occur throughout life. Various interventions and treatment options are available, depending on the specific traumatic injury sustained, but the fact is, every trauma is a unique case, which requires unique diagnosis and treatment.

The International Association of Dental Traumatology reports that one of every two children sustains a dental injury, most often between the ages of 8 and 12 years. The suggestion is in most cases of dental trauma; a rapid and appropriate intervention can lessen its impact from both oral and esthetic standpoint. To that end, the association has developed guidelines for the evaluation and management of traumatic dental injuries.

Although the oral region comprises a small part as 1% of the total body area, 5% of all bodily injuries are oral traumatic injuries. Traumatic dental injuries tend to occur at childhood or an young age during which growth and development take place. In preschool children, with injuries to the head being the most common, oral injuries make up as much as 17% of all bodily injuries, in contrast to later in life when injuries to hands and feet are the most common.

Dental injuries are the most common and are seen in as many as 92% of all patients seeking consultation or treatment for injuries to the oral region. Also, soft-tissue injuries are seen in 28%, simultaneously with dental injuries, and fractures involving the jaw are seen more rarely, in only 6% of all patients presenting with oral injuries [1–8].

Trauma has a multitude of consequences for the traumatized individual, family members, and society. The impact is not only physical but also psychosocial and economic. Every pediatric patient should be given the opportunity to receive a complete dental treatment for traumatic dental injuries, but a complete treatment plan involving participation of specialists in several disciplines can often be complicated and expensive. In contrast to many other traumatic injuries treated on an outpatient basis, traumatic dental injuries are mostly irreversible, and thus, treatment will likely continue for the rest of the patient's life [9–14].

Constructing a complete treatment plan can be challenging because of the diversity of evidence-based interventions and reported outcomes in clinical studies. Besides, there is evidence that clinical researchers may prefer reporting outcomes that enhance results—this is known as outcome reporting bias. International Association for Dental Traumatology suggests that this diversity and reporting bias shall be eliminated by a standardized trauma management guideline in order to make the outcomes relevant to patients, clinicians, and policy makers as findings of research are to influence practice and future research [15].

It has been reported that, anterior teeth, especially the maxillary central and lateral incisors are predominantly affected by traumatic dental injuries for both primary and permanent dentitions. Traumatic dental injuries generally affect a single tooth except certain trauma events, such as traffic accidents, violence, and sports injuries, which result in multiple tooth damage.

Besides its numerous beneficial effects, active participation in sports activities may increase the risk for traumatic injuries to oral and dental tissues. These injuries are most prominent in boxing, basketball, hockey, and soccer.

Traumatic dental injuries in the primary dentition appear to be rather stable at approximately 30% in most studies. It is been reported that one-third of all preschool children have suffered from traumatic injuries to the primary dentition in most of the countries. Although variations were observed within and between countries, one-fourth of all school children and almost one-third of adults have also suffered traumatic injuries to the permanent dentition [16–19].

2. Incidence and prevalence of dental trauma

The prevalence of dental injuries varies within countries regarding the research reports. According to two surveys in US, the prevalence of traumatic dental injuries varies between 18.4 and 16% in 6–20 years old and 27.1 and 28.1% in 21–50 years old age groups. In UK, dental trauma prevalence varies between 23.7 and 44.2% in 11–14-year age groups and mostly observed in schools [20–23]. In other European countries, the prevalence varies between 13.5 and 20.3% in 6–24-year age groups. In Middle East and Asia, the prevalence varies between 16.2 and 32% in 8–16 years old age groups as the 10–11 years age groups revealed the highest score. There is an absolute need for an international standardized trauma registration either being able to detect trends over time or to make reasonable comparisons between and within countries [24–32].

In most studies, it is been reported that the incidence of traumatic dental injuries in children shows a range of 1–3% in the population. The peak incidence for traumatic dental injuries per 1000 individuals is found up to 12 years of age. The incidence is lower in older ages. Boys are more often affected than girls.

The variation of both prevalence and incidence presented in the literature reflects the local differences, environmental variations, behavioral, cultural, and socioeconomic diversities as well as the lack of standardization in methods and classifications [12, 16, 33].

2.1 Etiologic risk factors

Etiologic factors are very much related to the age, gender, environment, and activity of the patient.

Age is an important factor, as school children and adolescent are the main groups who are mostly prone to traumatic injuries. It is estimated that 71–92% of all traumatic dental injuries occur before the age of 19 years; other studies have reported a decrease after the age of 24–30 years.

While in preschool children, the most common cause of traumatic dental injuries are accidental falls, in school age children, injuries are often caused by sports activities or hits by another person. Traffic accidents and assaults are the predominant etiologic factors in adolescents and young adults, and oral injuries occur most frequently during leisure time and during weekends associated with the western lifestyle today.

Gender is also a risk factor as males experience traumatic dental injuries at least twice more often than females. Yet, recent studies have shown a reduction in this gender difference in sports, which might be due to an increased interest in sports among girls Traebert et al. reported that girls can be exposed to the same risk factors of TDI as boys, which is a characteristic of modern Western society. Thus, environment and the activities of a person are undoubtedly more determining factors of TDIs than gender.

Another factor to be pointed is that in many countries, an increasing number of old people are possessing their own teeth, which, in near future, may lead to the increase in prevalence of dental traumatic injuries due to accidental falls in geriatric population [16, 33–35].

3. Guideline on management of acute dental trauma

3.1 Examination

Before making a treatment in trauma cases, dentist must check the circumstances written in below:

1. Patient's name, age, gender (include weight for young patients), address, and contact numbers

2. Symptoms of central nervous system should be checked after the accident

3. General health of the patient

4. Three W′ s must be asked "when, where, and how the injury occurred"

5. Treatment the patient received elsewhere

6. Previous dental injury history

7. Disturbances in the bite

8. Tooth reactions to thermal changes or sensitivity to sweet/sour
9. Soreness of the teeth during eating or by touching
10. If the patient is feeling spontaneous pain in the teeth.

Access for risk of concussion or hemorrhage:

- Symptoms may be delayed for minutes to hours
- It must be asked if there is a loss of consciousness
- Difficulty of speech and /or slurred speech
- Nausea/vomiting
- Fluid from ear/nose
- Confusion of situations
- Blurring in vision or uneven pupils.

3.2 History

- Timing
- Mechanism of injury
- Location
- Bleeding must be checked. Also, previous dental traumas should be asked.

3.3 Examination

Clinical examination consists of visual inspection, palpation, thermal testing, and electric pulp testing. First and foremost, account for all teeth:

- Extent of injury
- Lacerations
- Teeth position
- Appearance of tissue should be tested along with the color of tooth (purple, blue, gray, or yellow) and its mobility
- Pulp testing (percussion, EPT, and thermal): but if the traumatized tooth is immature, EPT may not be accurate
- Palpation of soft tissue must be recorded. Because the recordings will help you for follow-up appointments. Taking photographs may help to make proper

examination and diagnosis. These views are going to help the comparison of preoperative and follow-up of traumatized teeth.

3.4 Radiographs: AAE-recommended guidelines

- Occlusal
- Periapicals radiographs with different lateral angulations
- CBCT if more serious of an injury.

3.4.1 Panorex

- Periapical-radiographs taken from the same angle every time will help to make good treatment decisions. Using a film holder will hold the radiograph in a paralleling technique
- Occlusal
- CBCT.

3.5 Types of dental trauma on hard tissue and pulp

Enamel infraction
Enamel fracture
Enamel-dentin fracture
Enamel-dentin-pulp fracture
Crown-root fracture w/o pulp involvement
Crown-root fracture with pulp involvement.

3.6 Types of dental trauma on periodontal tissue

Concussion
Subluxation (loosening)
Intrusive luxation (central dislocation)
Extrusive luxation (partial avulsion)
Lateral luxation
Retained root fracture.

3.7 Types of dental trauma on supporting bone

Exarticulation (complete avulsion)
Comminution of the alveolar socket
Alveolar socket wall fracture
Alveolar process fracture
Mandible or maxilla fracture.

3.8 Types of dental trauma on gingival or oral mucosa

Gingival or oral mucosal laceration
Gingival or oral mucosal contusion
Gingival or oral mucosal abrasion (**Figures 1–3**) [9, 11–13, 15, 36, 37].

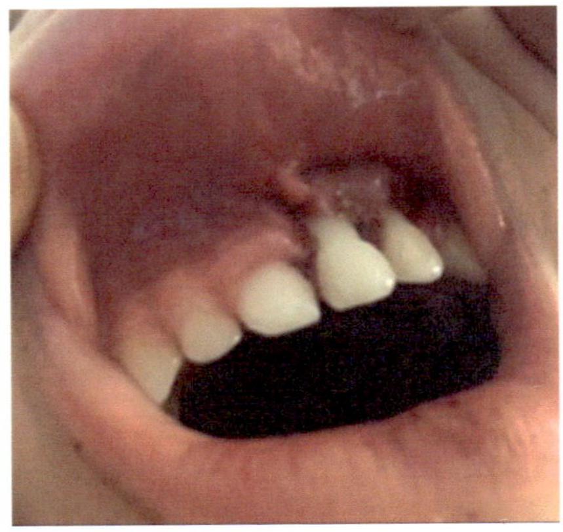

Figure 1.
Types of dental trauma: gingival laceration.

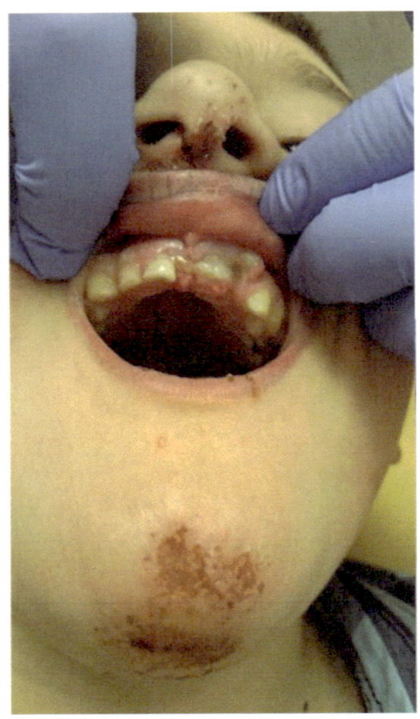

Figure 2.
Types of dental trauma: intrusive luxation (central dislocation).

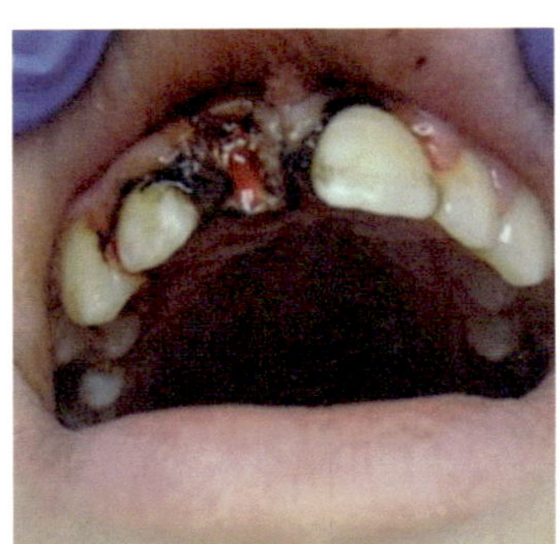

Figure 3.
Types of dental trauma: crown-root fracture with pulp involvement.

4. Dental trauma in primary dentition

Pain treatment and prevention of teeth germs must be our main goal in the treatment strategy of the traumatized primary teeth. Due to behavioral management problems or a severe trauma with a soft tissue bleeding, treatment may be overlooked or limited to extraction. However, in the overall treatment, primary teeth must be followed up clinically and radiographically in the long term.

In this section, treatment of primary dentition will be explained based on IADT treatment guidelines.

Enamel fracture: this type of fracture involves only enamel. There is no radiographic abnormality observed. Sharp edges are recommended to be smoothened. There is no need for follow-up.

Enamel dentin fracture: fracture involves enamel and dentin. Pulp is not exposed. There is no radiographic abnormality observed. The relation between the fracture and the pulp chamber can be revealed. In case behavioral management is succeeded with the patient, involved dentin can be sealed completely with glass ionomer to prevent microleakage. Composite resin restorations are good choices if lost tooth structure is large. Clinical examination is required after 3–4 weeks.

Crown fracture with exposed pulp: fracture involves enamel and dentin and the pulp is exposed. Radiographic findings can reveal the stage of root development. Preservation of pulp vitality can be accomplished by partial pulpotomy. Unless there is an cooperation with the patient, extraction is an alternative treatment approach. Clinical follow-up is required after 1 week, 6–8 weeks, and 1 year. Radiographic follow-up is required after 6–8 weeks and 1 year as well (**Figure 4**).

Crown/root fracture (without pulp exposure): this type of fracture involves enamel, dentin, and root structure. The pulp may or may not be exposed. Tooth displacement may be observed as well. Radiographical evaluation will reveal single/multiple fragments of the traumatized tooth. In case the fracture involves only a small part of the root, only fractured fragment is removed and coronal restoration can be done if the stable fragment is adequate for restoration. Otherwise, extraction is required. Clinical follow-up is required after 1 week, 6–8 weeks, and 1 year. Radiographic follow-up is required after 6–8 weeks and 1 year as well. Monitoring is vital until eruption of the successors.

Crown/root fracture (with pulp exposure): this type of fracture involves enamel and dentin and the pulp is exposed. The stage of development of root can be determined by the radiographic evaluation. Preservation of pulp vitality can be accomplished by partial pulpotomy using calcium hydroxide paste and reinforced

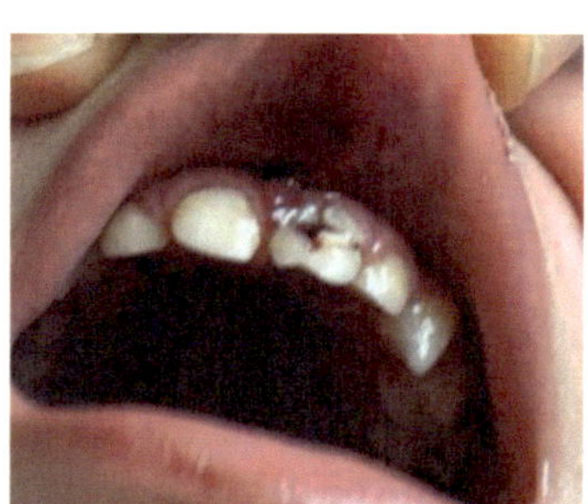

Figure 4.
Crown fracture in primary dentition.

glass ionomer as liner and composite/compomer restorations. Unless there is a co-operation with the patient, extraction is an alternative treatment approach. Clinical follow-up is required after 1 week, 6–8 weeks, and 1 year. Radiographic follow-up is required after 6–8 weeks and 1 year as well.

Root fracture: the fracture involves the alveolar bone and may extend to adjacent bone leading to segment mobility and dislocation. Frequently, an occlusal interference is reported. Radiographic evaluation is required to assess the fracture line position. Treatment should be repositioning the displaced segment and splinting. Stabilization must be for 4 weeks. Monitoring the fracture line is essential. If there is no displacement, 1 week, 6–8 weeks, and 1 year clinical follow-up are required. After 1 year, radiographic evaluation should be repeated until eruption of the successors. If the traumatized tooth/teeth are extracted as treatment choice after 1 year, both clinical and radiographic examination are still required for monitoring successors.

Alveolar fracture: the tooth is displaced, usually in a palatal/lingual or labial direction leading to mobility. Occlusal radiographic findings will reveal increased periodontal ligament space apically at its best. If there is no occlusal interference, the tooth is allowed to reposition spontaneously. If there is minor occlusal interference, slight grinding is indicated. When there is more severe occlusal interference, the tooth can be gently repositioned by combined labial and palatal pressure after the use of local anesthesia. In severe cases, when the crown is dislocated in a labial direction, extraction is indicated. Follow-ups are required as follows: 1 week and 2–3 weeks of clinical examination, and 6–8 weeks and 1 year clinical and radiographic examinations.

Concussion: clinically, tooth is sensitive to touch. There is no mobility or sulcular bleeding observed. Radiographic evaluation discloses no pathology as well. Observation is the only treatment option. Only clinical follow-up is required after 1 and 6–8 weeks.

Subluxation: an increased mobility is observed though the tooth is not displaced. There might be cervical bleeding. There is no abnormality in the radiographic evaluation. Occlusal radiography can screen possible root fracture and displacement. Observation is the only treatment option. Soft brushing and use of antibacterial agents is recommended. Only clinical follow-up is required after 1 and 6–8 weeks. Parents should be informed about an occurrence of possible crown discoloration. Unless a fistula is formed, monitoring is required.

Extrusive luxation: the tooth appears elongated due to its displacement out of its socket. Thus, it can be excessively mobile. Increased apical periodontal ligament space is disclosed in radiographic evaluation. For minor extrusion (<3 mm) in an immature developing tooth, careful repositioning or leaving the tooth for spontaneous alignment can be the treatment options. Extraction is indicated for severe extrusion in a fully formed primary tooth. Clinical follow-up is required after 1 week, 6–8 weeks, and 1 year. Radiographic follow-up is required after 6–8 weeks and 1 year as well. Parents should be informed about the possible occurrence of discoloration.

Lateral luxation: the tooth is displaced, usually in a palatal/lingual or labial direction and will be immobile. If there is no occlusal interference, the tooth is allowed to reposition spontaneously. For minor occlusal interference, slight grinding is indicated. If there is more severe occlusal interference, the tooth can be gently repositioned after the use of local anesthesia. If the crown is dislocated severely in a labial direction, extraction is indicated. Clinical follow-up is required after 1 week, 6–8 weeks, and 1 year. Radiographic follow-up is required after 6–8 weeks and 1 year as well.

Intrusive luxation: when the apex is displaced toward labial bone plate, the apical tip appears shorter than its contra lateral and the tooth is left for spontaneous repositioning. When the apex is displaced toward the permanent tooth germ, tooth appears elongated and must be extracted. Clinical follow-ups are required for 1 week, 3–4 weeks, 6–8 weeks, 6 months, and 1 year after, whereas radiographic follow-up is 6–8 weeks and 1 year later. Clinical and radiographic monitoring is essential until eruption of the permanent successor.

Avulsion: clinical findings reveal that tooth is not in the socket; however, radiographic examination is required to confirm and not to overlook intrusion. Replantation of the avulsed teeth is not recommended. Clinical follow-ups are required for 1 week, 6 months, and 1 year after, whereas radiographic follow-up is for 6 months and 1 year after to monitor successors' eruption.

5. Classification, definition, examination, and treatment planning in dental traumas

5.1 Hard tissue and pulp in permanent dentition

Enamel infraction: no need to restore.

Enamel-fracture: it is a kind of uncomplicated crown fracture. An enamel fracture is a crown fracture limited to loss of enamel only. Small enamel fractures can be polished. Composite resin restoration may be preferred for more involved enamel fractures (**Figure 5**).

Enamel-dentin fracture: it is a kind of uncomplicated crown fracture. The tooth should be restored with composite resin. If the fragment is available, reattachment of fragment can be attempted (**Figure 6**).

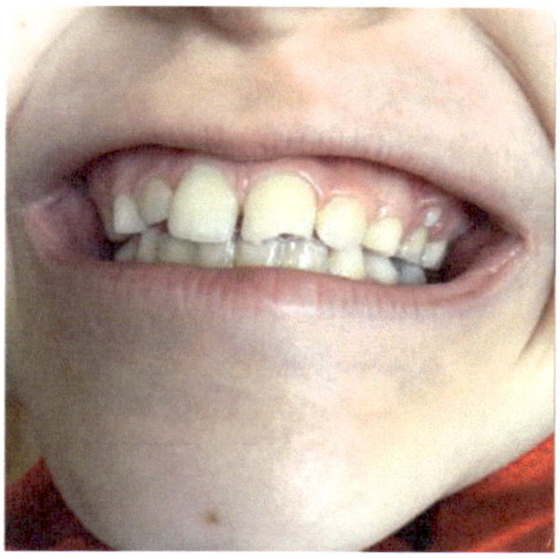

Figure 5.
Enamel fracture.

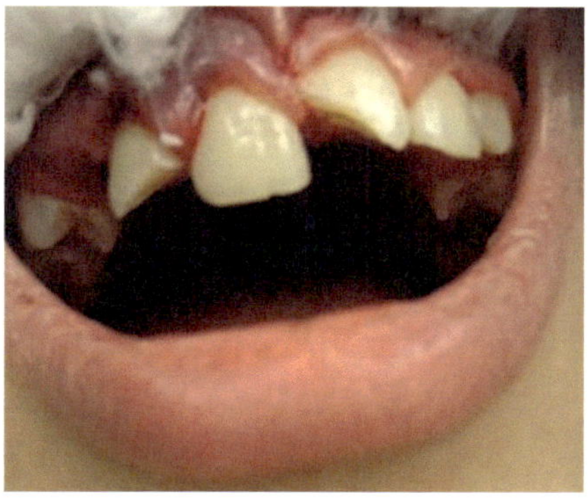

Figure 6.
Enamel-dentin and pulp fracture.

Enamel-dentin-pulp fracture: a complicated crown fracture involves enamel and dentin with pulp exposure. If the pulp exposure is visible, only a pink spot or bluish exposure site is cleaned and pulp-capping agent is applied. For larger pulpal exposures, partial pulpotomy and direct pulp-capping procedures are performed. Crown restoration method is the same as in uncomplicated crown fractures. Pulp capping and restoration should be performed at the same appointment, if possible (**Figures 6–8**).

Crown fracture combined with luxation results in ischemic changes that can lead to pulp necrosis. In these cases, there is no response to vitality tests. It is possible that the tooth has sustained a luxation injury and pulp necrosis (coagulation necrosis) is present. According to Dr. Tsukiboshi, for young patients under 18 years of age, regardless of pulp vitality, the restoration of the tooth should be done. Then, the patient should be followed for 1, 3, and 6 months to determine pulp vitality. After the waiting period, if pulp necrosis occurs, root canal treatment needs to be performed. Adult patients with a traumatized mature tooth with closed apex, after the confirmation of pulp necrosis in the first appointment, root canal treatment should be completed. Otherwise, pulpectomy may be performed (**Figures 9** and **10**).

Crown-root fracture w/o pulp involvement: the treatment is similar to the uncomplicated crown fracture. Firstly, necessity of pulp capping or partial pulpotomy is evaluated and then, rearrangement of the fragment is performed. If no need to pulp capping or partial pulpotomy, flowable composite resin may help to combine the fractured parts of the crown.

Crown-root fracture with pulp involvement: in these cases, the fractured segment accounts for the larger part of the crown and the fracture line has extended to the alveolar crest or below. These teeth may be seen too difficult to restore, but the location of the fracture line may help to decide the treatment procedure. If the location of the fracture line is located within the coronal third of the root, crown restoration is possible after the extrusion of the root. There are two ways for extrusion of the root: orthodontic or surgical.

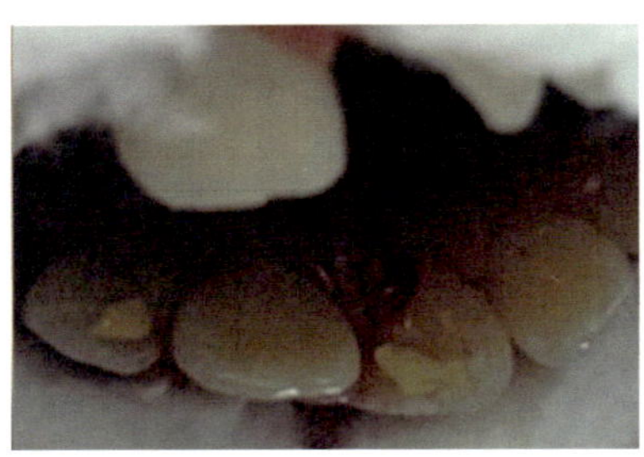

Figure 7.
Pulp capping after dental trauma.

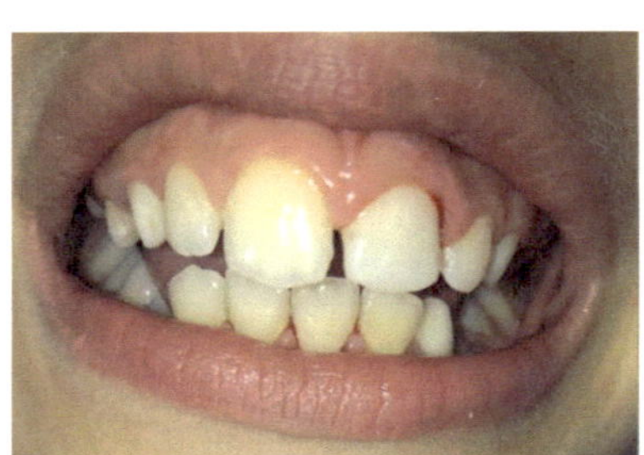

Figure 8.
Restoration during first appointment.

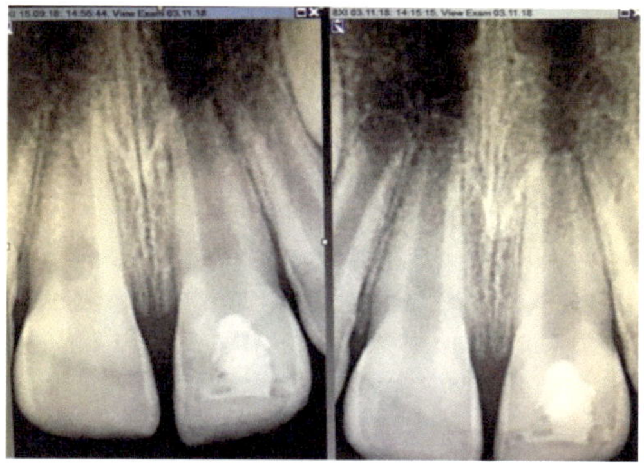

Figure 9.
Young patient's traumatized teeth with open apex.

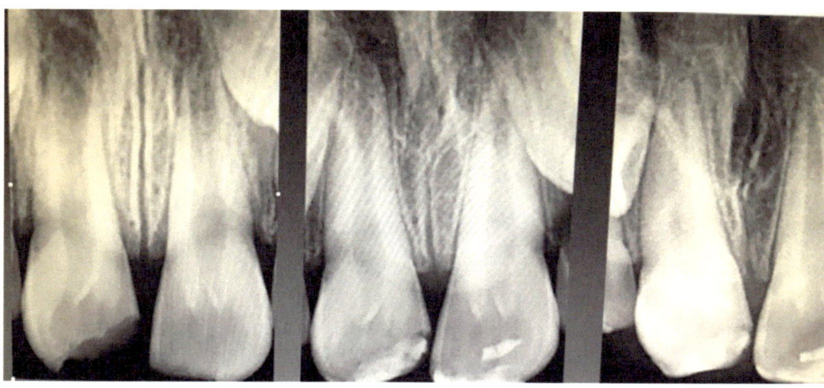

Figure 10.
Closure of apex of traumatized incisor after 1.5 years.

5.2 Root fracture

Root fracture is a fracture that involves cementum, dentin, and pulp. The fracture line may be horizontal, oblique, or vertical. But vertical root fractures may generally occur in endodontically treated teeth. For that reason, in this chapter, horizontally or obliquely fractured teeth will be considered.

Root fractures are classified as shallow or deep according to the location of fracture line. Root fracture is generally diagnosed by radiographs. Sometimes, displacement of the coronal segment is not present. So, the fracture line is easily missed by conventional radiographic techniques. Therefore, it is better to take the radiograph from different angles. Or cone beam computed tomography may be used to diagnose the root fractures. Otherwise, fracture lines may be discovered after several months.

While performing electric pulp testing, tooth may not be responding to it. In that cases, three possibilities may be thought: pulp tissue is severed at the fracture, there is no severance of the pulp, only the subluxation in the apical fragment or the pulp is severed, and the apical fragment is subluxated.

5.2.1 Treatment planning of deep root fractures

The treatment of deep root fracture is simple: repositioning and fixation of coronal segment. Depending on how deep the fracture is and how mobile the coronal segment is, fixation may be required for up to 3 months. Six months later, if there is no pulp necrosis, there will be no need to root canal treatment. In case of pulp necrosis, root canal treatment is done up to the fracture line [9, 10, 36–39].

5.2.2 Treatment planning of shallow root fractures

Restorative treatment can be very difficult. Sometimes extraction is the best treatment planning. If the extraction is the chosen treatment, the patient's age, oral condition, oral hygiene habits, the tooth's position, and the occlusion should be evaluated and then autotransplantation may be considered as an alternative plan.

5.3 Subluxation

Subluxation is clinically defined as injury to the periodontal tissues accompanied by bleeding from gingival sulcus, an increase in mobility but no dislocation of the tooth. There is sensitivity in percussion, and high mobility and bleeding are important criteria in diagnosis of subluxation. Electric pulp testing is important. In immature tooth, electric pulp testing will not respond, so re-test with electric pulp testing after a week is advised.

5.3.1 Treatment planning

In immature tooth: only follow-up is necessary. Root canal treatment is indicated in the presence of pulp necrosis. When there is a possibility of pulp necrosis, root canal treatment can be initiated without anesthesia.

In mature tooth: follow-up visits without invasive treatment are advised 6–12 months after injury to allow pulp vitality to be recovered. In case of pulp necrosis, root canal treatment is indicated.

5.4 Extrusive luxation

Extrusive luxation results in damage to the periodontal tissues as the tooth is displaced in coronal direction. The periodontal tissue and the root are not completely separated, but the blood supply at the apex is disrupted. There is high mobility, bleeding, and electric pulp testing response is negative. Radiographically, there is widening in periodontal ligament space.

5.4.1 Treatment planning

Repositioning, fixation, and follow-up are the steps of treatment planning. Root canal treatment is avoided until pulp necrosis is confirmed. After confirmation of pulp necrosis, root canal treatment is indicated. In ımmature tooth, apexification and apexogenesis may be applicable.

5.5 Lateral luxation

Lateral luxation is an injury to the periodontal and alveolar supporting tissues that the tooth displaces laterally. The crown of the tooth is displaced palatally or lingually, and the tooth may be apically displaced with alveolar bone fracture on the labial side. The blood supply is completely disrupted at the apical side, but periodontal tissues have not been separated. Radiographically, the root shape and alveolar socket are not aligned. Sometimes, the traumatized teeth may be locked because of fracture on alveolar bone. This situation may be confused with ankylosis.

5.5.1 Treatment planning

Repositioning, fixation, and regular follow-up are the steps of treatment of lateral luxation. In fixation period, if alveolar fracture occurs, fixation period will take at least 3 months. Root canal treatment may be delayed until pulp necrosis has been confirmed. In young adults, apexification and apexogenesis may be treatment alternatives (**Figures 11** and **12**).

5.6 Intrusive luxation

Intrusion is a luxation injury that results in apical displacement of tooth. In some cases, alveolar bone fracture is also seen. In the diagnosis of ıntrusion, differential

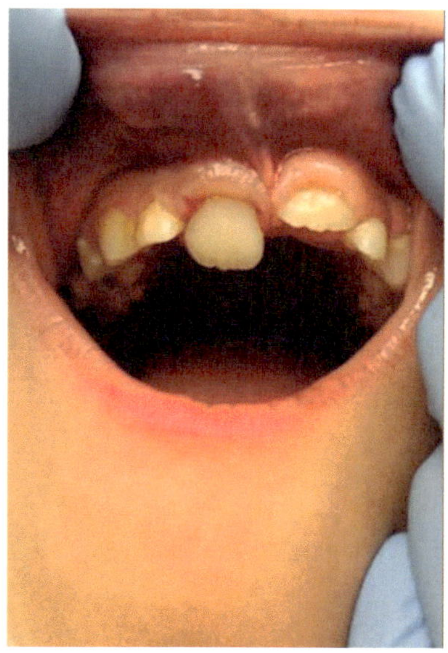

Figure 11.
Lateral luxated central incisor.

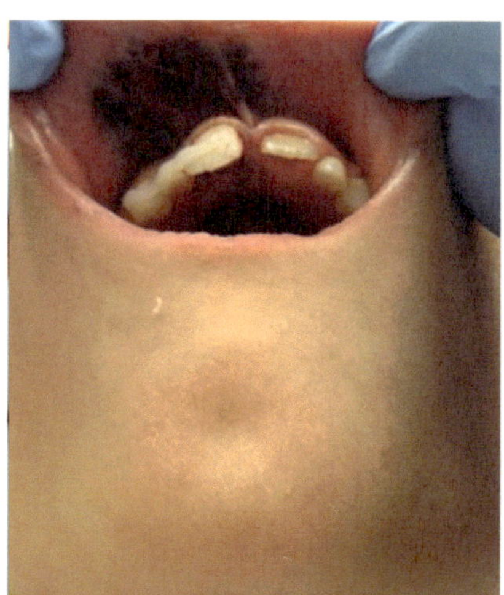

Figure 12.
Splinting after lateral luxation.

diagnostic criteria should be detected. If the tooth is intruded apically compared with adjacent teeth, intrusion should be thought. Reduced mobility may also be seen. Percussion sound is a metallic sound. There is no percussion sensitivity. If there is no clear periodontal ligament in radiograph, the intrusion should be suspected. CBCT images are important to differentiate the diagnosis of lateral or intrusive luxation (**Figure 13**).

5.6.1 Treatment planning

The healing of intruded tooth may be affected by some factors such as patient's age, root development degree, and depth of intrusion.

According to some studies, as age increases, the incidence of pulp necrosis, loss of marginal bone, and root resorption also increase. If intrusion is more than 7 mm, the more complications may be seen compared with those that are intruded less than 3 mm. Time between injury and treatment, type of fixation, and use of antibiotics may also affect the results.

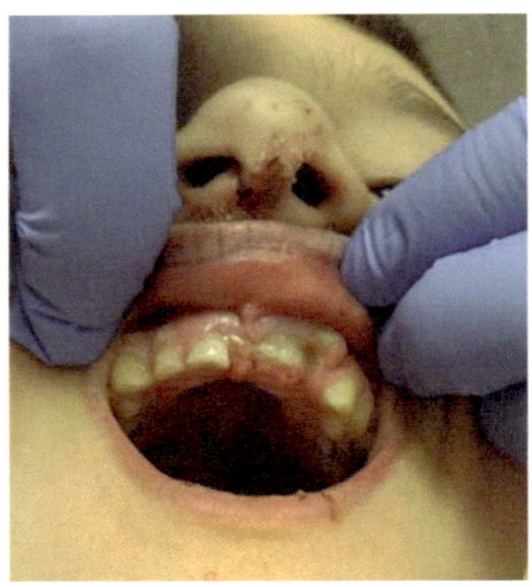

Figure 13.
An intruded central incisor.

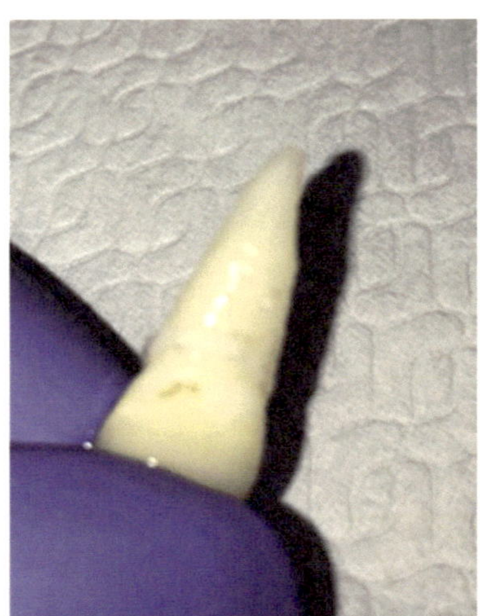

Figure 14.
An avulsed tooth.

Spontaneous re-eruption, orthodontic extrusion, and the surgical extrusion are the main options of intrusive luxation.

Dr. Tsukiboshim suggests spontaneous re-eruption when the depth of intrusion is shallow and the root is immature whereas surgical extrusion is indicated when the depth of intrusion is deep and the root is mature.

5.7 Transient apical breakdown (TAB)

TAB is a phenomenon linked to the repair processes in the traumatized pulp or pulp and periodontium of luxated mature teeth, which returns to normal when repair is completed. This phenomenon is described by Frances Andreasen in 1986.

5.8 Avulsion

Avulsion is defined as the condition that the whole tooth is completely separated from the supporting tissues.

The success rate for an avulsed tooth after replantation depends on the vitality of periodontal ligament and attachment of the tooth (**Figure 14**) [9–12, 15, 24, 26, 27, 31, 36–40].

6. Splinting

6.1 A splint may be necessary to stabilize the traumatized tooth after injury

Dental splint is a rigid or flexible device or compound used to support, protect, or immobilize teeth that have been loosened, replanted, fractured, or subjected to certain endodontic surgical procedures (**Figures 15–17**).

6.1.1 Flexible splinting assists in healing

Characteristics of the ideal splint include:

1. easy to fabricate in the mouth and without extra trauma to the tooth
2. passive if not orthodontic forces are intended
3. allows for physiologic mobility
4. nonirritant to soft tissues, periodontal tissues, and noncarcinogenic
5. does not interfere with occlusion
6. easy to permit endodontic access and vitality testing
7. easy to clean
8. easy to remove
9. allows for pulp testing and endodontic treatments
10. relatively inexpensive

11. provides patient comfort and esthetic appearance

12. easily accessible and easy to maintain oral hygiene.

6.1.2 Types of splints

Rigid splints: are used in cervical root fractures and alveolar bone fractures. Stainless steel wire >0.5 mm, direct composite resin or titanium ring splint (TTS), or direct composite resin reinforced with fiberglass ribbon can be used.

Flexible splints: allow for optimal pulp and periodontal ligament healing. Nylon, stainless steel wire <0.4 mm, nickel titanium wires up to 0.016 with composite resin, and glass ionomer cement splints are used.

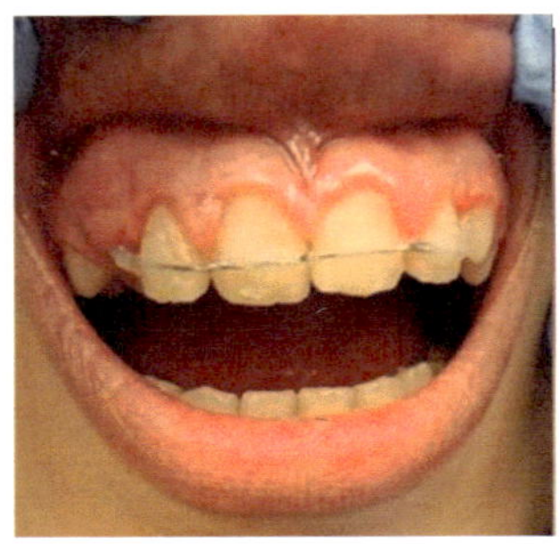

Figure 15.
Splint with ligature wire.

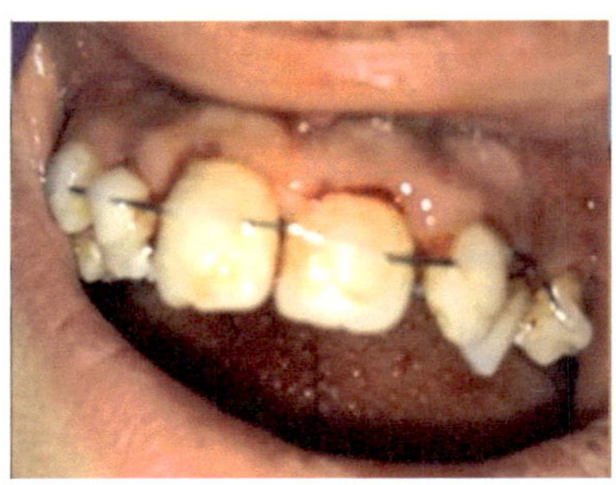

Figure 16.
Arch wire and composite splint.

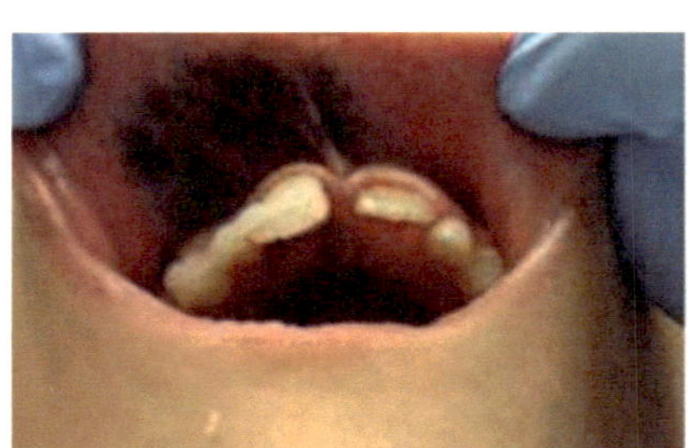

Figure 17.
Composite resin splint.

Compound splints: orthodontic bracket and wire are used as compound splint materials.

Instructions to patients having a splint placed include to:

1. taking a soft diet

2. avoid eating on teeth having splint

3. maintain a detailed oral hygiene

4. use chlorhexidine/antibiotics if prescribed

5. reach the dental office immediately if splint breaks/loosens.

Before beginning or continuing orthodontic treatment, traumatized teeth must be checked carefully.

It is recommended that even if there is a minor trauma to the teeth, one should wait for at least 3 months for orthodontic movement. Any kind of dental traumas to hard or soft dental tissues (e.g., minor concussions, subluxations, and extrusions) also requires a 3-month waiting period. For moderate to severe trauma/damage to the periodontium, at least 6 months of waiting period is recommended.

In root fracture cases, the tooth must not be moved for at least 1 year. If there is radiographic evidence of healing, those teeth may be moved successfully [15, 36–39].

7. Regenerative endodontic treatment of necrotic immature permanent teeth due to dental trauma

An immature permanent tooth is defined by the British Society of Pediatric Dentistry as a tooth that is not fully formed, particularly the root apex. A vital pulp is necessary for the development and maturation of the tooth root [40]. Completion of the root development of the teeth and closure of the root apex takes place 2–3 years after the eruption of the teeth. If pulp necrosis occurs for any reason (trauma, caries, etc.) before root development is complete, the root development undergoes a standstill, so the root remains without closure. In such cases, root canal treatment is both inevitable and difficult to do, because the root canal is very large, and the dentin walls are very thin and fragile [16, 40–43].

As a result of trauma, opening of the pulp tissue into the oral cavity may lead to infection by reaching the pulp tissue of oral microorganisms [44]. However, damage to the vascular nerve pack at the apex of the severely traumatized tooth causes necrosis of pulp tissue [41, 44].

The completion of the root formation of immature teeth that have necrotic pulp, or the induction of a calcified barrier formation at the root apices is defined as apexification [21].

There are various difficulties in the treatment of immature necrosed young permanent teeth:

- the difficulty of cleaning and shaping the canals

- difficulty of canal disinfection

- the risk of breakage of thin fragile dentin walls during mechanical obturation

- short crown/root ratio
- material carried out of the apex
- it is difficult or impossible to perform a possible retreatment in the future due to thin canal walls.

Until now, two apexification procedures for these teeth have been performed successfully. First of these procedures is conventional apexification inducing the formation of a barrier to apical calcification using calcium dihydroxide. Second is a one-step apexification method that provides production of an artificial apical barrier using mineral trioxide aggregate (MTA). In both the methods, constriction of apical foramen of an immature tooth has been shown [16, 38, 42, 43].

Traditional apexification treatment requires a large number of sessions, and problems with patient compliance may occur. Long-term use of calcium hydroxide may lead changing physical properties of dentin.

As a result of requirements of short-term completion of canal treatments, acceleration of healing and reduction of the sessions was sought response to one-step apexification with apex closuring by using MTA that has been on the agenda [25].

Advantages of MTA apexification over calcium hydroxide apexification are more such as reliable barrier formation, reduction in treatment time, requirement of lesser visits, hence reducing the root fractures and preventing the changing of physical properties of dentin. In addition, since the MTA is not cytotoxic, its biological properties are advantageous and induce tissue repair.

Despite the popularity among clinicians, there are disadvantages of the apexification technique compared with MTA:

- the inability to control the applied condensation pressure and increased risk of fracture of thin dentin walls at large pressures
- it is difficult to remove after hardening, and surgical methods are needed for removing
- the high alkalinity of the material affects the stiffness of the root dentin over time
- high cost
- short shelf-life
- the challenges of clinical practice.

However, the risk of development of cervical root fractures remains high after apexification treatments [28].

The disadvantages of traditional apexification treatments have led the researchers to quest an alternative treatment approach that restores the function of the pulp dentin complex and persists its development. This quest led to arise of regeneration and regenerative endodontic treatment.

In biology dictionaries, regeneration is defined as the regrowth by an animal or plant of an organ, tissue, or part that has been lost or destroyed [21].

Regenerative endodontics is one of the most exciting new developments in endodontics. The current (2016) American Association of Endodontists' Glossary of Endodontic Terms defines regenerative endodontics as "biologically-based procedures designed to physiologically replace damaged tooth structures, including dentin and root structures, as well as cells of the pulp-dentin complex" [21].

Regenerative endodontic procedures, a new approach to preventing tooth loss, aim to restore the damaged pulp and dentin structures, create a new pulp tissue in the canal, and provide root maturation [16, 28, 38, 43].

Seeking to find the ideal treatment method within the regenerative endodontics continues. The most studied methods in this area are: root canal revascularization, stem cell therapy, pulp implants, scaffold implants, injectable scaffold applications, three-dimensional cell software, and gene therapy. However, only the root canal revascularization could be used clinically in the treatment of traumatized necrotic young permanent teeth [28].

Revascularization term is used to indicate the restoration of blood flow to the necrotic pulp cavity. Despite the fact that pulpless teeth can sustain their presence in the mouth for a long time after successful endodontic treatment, the viability of the dental pulp offers many advantages, including the formation of reparative dentin, the completion of apical closure, and the development of dentin walls. Via the root canal revascularization, the pulp tissue is regenerated and the permanence of the tooth vitality is ensured [28, 38].

There are also negative aspects such as the fact that some dental pathologies, such as progressive decay, cannot be recognized by patients due to the loss of sensitivity to environmental changes by pulpless teeth.

In addition, the elimination of the negative consequences of traditional root canal treatment procedures is the reason why revascularization is preferred in the treatment of necrotic traumatized young permanent teeth.

At the basis of revascularization lies the rationale that "new cells can develop in the presence of sterile tissue matrix and pulp vitality can be restored," because when dental canal infection is under control, it becomes a necrotic, avulse tooth condition with sterile pulp cavity. Regeneration in the apical tissues after the avulsion and replantation suggests regeneration may occur in the pulp tissue of a necrotic and infected tooth [16, 43, 45].

In the revascularization method, after the necrotic root canal is totally disinfected, it is aimed to provide a fibrin matrix with the blood clot formed by the bleeding from the tooth apex provided by the over instrumentation. Revascularization is observed through the new cell development via the differentiation of few stem cells preserved vital, in this provided sterile matrix [16, 43].

Hargreaves et al. recommended three major components of pulp regeneration called triad of regenerative endodontics:

a. a dependable stem cell source that has capability of differentiating into odontoblasts

b. a suitable scaffold to support cell growth and differentiation, and

c. signaling molecules that have capability to stimulate cellular proliferation and direct cellular differentiation [28].

Stem cells are nondifferentiated cells that are capable of differentiating themselves into specialized cells, which can be transformed into many different cell types, when appropriate conditions are achieved within the body or in the laboratory. They are self-renewing and thus can generate any tissue for a lifetime unlike other progenitor cells [21].

Stem cell sources that play a role in the regeneration and root development of pulp tissue in the treatment of revascularization include dental pulp cells that maintain the viability of the root canal, stem cells originating from the apical papilla, and periodontal ligament [16, 19].

Blood clot is a very rich source of growth factors and has an important role in the differentiation, maturation, and regeneration of fibroblast, odontoblast, and cementoblast [23].

7.1 The importance of root canal disinfection in revascularization treatments

Absence of bacteria in the root canal is critical for successful revascularization therapy, because the development of new tissue stops when it encounters bacteria in the canal cavity.

The most effective root canal disinfection method is provided by drugs applied to the root canal in addition to chemical irrigation.

However, a good preparation in open apex tooth and the use of cytotoxic antiseptics may remove pulp cells that are well fed and viable in the apical region. Removal of these tissues means removal of cells with the potential to convert to pulp and dentin [16, 41, 43, 46].

Sato et al., who applied the triple antibiotic paste in vitro for the first time, reported that triple antibiotic paste is effective in the treatment of dentin infected by *Escherichia coli* [46].

7.2 Patient selection criteria for revascularization treatment

The success of the treatment is based on the right case selection. No studies have been conducted on the success of revascularization therapy in individuals with genetic disease, severe medical disease, or poor immune system. Therefore, revascularization therapy procedures should be limited to systemically healthy people.

Revascularization therapy is not suitable for individuals allergic to triple antibiotics used in the canal.

It is not indicated in patients who cannot adapt or participate in the treatment process due to being a long-term and follow-up procedure, and in individuals who are fearful or uncooperative [42, 45, 47].

7.3 Tooth selection criteria for revascularization treatment

First of all, the tooth to be treated should be necrosis. Other regenerative therapies are considered such as pulp capping or partial pulpotomy with regenerative medicaments in teeth with vital pulp and partial pulpitis.

The presence of radiolucency in the periapical region as well as vitality tests has long been used as a determining factor. In both cases, vital pulp cells and apical papilla can still be present in the canal and apex.

Another criterion is the presence of infection. However, as a hypothesis, the presence of long-term infection adversely affects the survival of the pulp tissue and stem cell continuity, and makes it difficult to control the infection.

Since apex opening greater than 1 mm increases success, it should be preferred in immature young permanent teeth. Although a very few researchers recommend to expand the apex with a hand piece in the teeth with closed apex having less than 1 mm apex opening, but in the guidelines, the indication is limited to the open apex teeth.

Furthermore, the loss of coronal tissue in the teeth that will be treated with revascularization should not exceed the size for allowing it to be restored, and tissue damage should not be large, requiring to be made post/core [16, 41–43, 47].

8. Procedures in regenerative endodontics

An informed consent document must be taken before the treatment. This document should include the informations of complications such as tooth coloration or treatment failure, side effects such as pain or infection that may be able to emerge, two (or more) appointments will be needed, and what type of antibiotics will be used. Also, besides the nontreatment option, the patient must be informed about the tooth extraction (when deemed the tooth is nonsalvageable), and calcium hydroxide and MTA apexifications as the alternative treatments of revascularization. Following the consent document signing, treatment can be commenced [16, 18, 19, 25, 28, 38, 41–44, 46–49].

8.1 First appointment

Under local anesthesia and rubber dam isolation, an access cavity is prepared for the treatment. Each root canal opening is expanded to facilitate the placement of the medicament. The remaining root canal is not instrumented.

Copious, passive irrigation is made with 20 ml of 1.5% sodium hypochlorite (NaOCl), for 5 minutes to each canal, followed by a sterile saline solution or EDTA (20 ml for each canal, 5 minutes). It is important to maintain the vitality of stem cells in the apical tissues. Therefore, an irrigation system such as needle with closed end and side vents is used to minimize the odds of extrusion of irrigant agents into the periapical area. Also, the irrigation needle should be positioned approximately 1 mm from the root end to minimize cytotoxicity to stem cells in the apical tissues.

After sufficient irrigation, the canals are gently dried with sterile paper points.

Calcium hydroxide, or low concentration of triple antibiotic paste, can be used to fill the canals.

A triple antibiotic paste is an antibiotic mix made from tablets of ciprofloxacin, metronidazole, and minocycline in a ratio of 1:1:1. For preparation, after removal of the coatings on the tablets, the tablets are pulverized and mixed in a 1:1:1 ratio in a sterile saline to form a paste-like consistency.

Triple antibiotic paste has been associated with tooth discoloration; therefore, if it is used, to minimize risk of staining, pulp chamber is sealed with a dentin bonding agent and ensure that it should remain below cemento-enamel junction (CEJ).

For minimizing the coronal staining, modified triple antibiotic paste obtained by adding another antibiotic (e.g., clindamycin, amoxicillin, and cefaclor) instead of minocycline, or minocycline-free double antibiotic pat, may also be used.

After delivering the paste into the canals via syringe, a sterile cotton pellet is placed into the canal below the CEJ and the cavity is sealed with temporary filling so as not to allow microleakage.

8.2 Second appointment (1–4 weeks after first visit)

In the second appointment, 1–4 weeks after the first visit, the response of the initial treatment is evaluated. If the clinical signs/symptoms persisted, the first appointment treatment procedures are repeated with antimicrobials, or alternative antimicrobials.

If the tooth has become asymptomatic, the second session is started through the anesthesia with 3% mepivacaine free of vasoconstrictor.

After the tooth is isolated with rubber dam, the temporary filling and cotton pellet are removed.

Following the removing of the paste from the canals by irrigation with 20 ml of 17% EDTA, the canals are dried with sterile paper points.

Bleeding into canal system to the level of CEJ is created by 2 mm over-instrumenting through rotating a precurved K-file. The using of platelet-rich plasma (PRP), platelet-rich fibrin (PRF), or autologous fibrin matrix (AFM) has been considered as the alternatives to create a blood clot, especially when bleeding into the canal cannot be achieved.

Bleeding is stopped at a level allowing for 3–4 mm of restorative material. In order to ensure the formation of blood clot, place a sterile cotton pellet for 3–4 minutes upon the bleeding. If it is necessary, placing a resorbable matrix (e.g., CollaPlug™, Collacote™, and CollaTape™) over the blood clot is applicable.

For stabilizing the white MTA that is used as a capping material, 3–4 mm layer of light-curing glass ionomer is flowed gently over it. Because the MTA has been associated with discoloration, it should be placed just below the level of the CEJ, over the blood clot. If there is an esthetic concern, alternative materials of MTA like bioceramics or tricalcium silicate cements should be considered.

Finally, the access cavity is restored with a suitable restorative material [16, 18, 19, 25, 28, 38, 41–44, 46–49].

8.3 MTA as a coating material

MTA, with quite good physical properties in terms of covering and sealing, is one of the most ideal coating materials to be used for the hermeticity of coronary closure.

In addition, the application with glass ionomer resin increases its covering properties and durability.

To allow more root growth, the MTA should be 1–2 mm thick below the CEJ.

Placing the MTA on the formed clot is a technically difficult procedure. Care should be taken during condensation, because the material can be moved from the CEJ to the apical point [16, 43].

8.4 Follow-up, goals, and success in revascularization treatment

Appointments are given to the patient at intervals of 3–6 months, and root formation is monitored clinically and radiographically.

The success of pulp revascularization treatment depends on three elements: root canal disinfection, the presence of a scaffold (blood clot), and hermetic coronary filling [38, 45].

The degree of success of regenerative endodontic procedures is largely measured by the degree to which primary, secondary and tertiary goals are achieved.

Primary goal: elimination of symptoms and healing of bone tissue.

Secondary goal: the increase in the thickness and/or the length of the root walls (although it is a desirable condition).

Tertiary goal: positive response to vitality test (indicates the presence of a more organized vital pulp tissue).

Five different types of responses to revascularization treatments are available:

Type 1—thickening and root development of canal walls

Type 2—the root of the root end is blunt and closed and the root growth is stopped

Type 3—root development continues, but the apex remains open

Type 4—common calcification in canal cavity

Type 5—hard tissue barrier formation between root apex and coronal MTA.

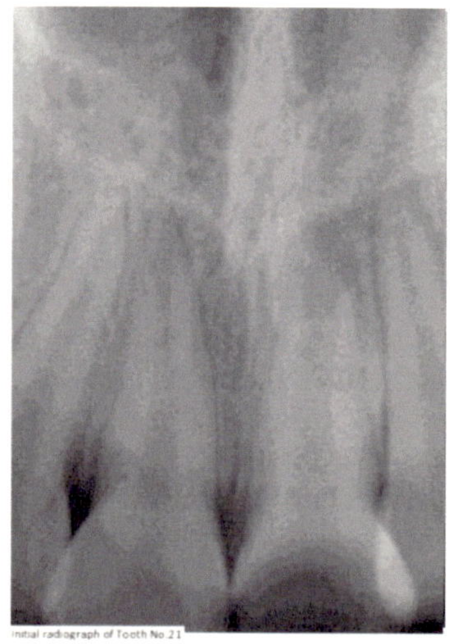

Figure 18.
A necrotic, immature, 21 numbered teeth, due to dental trauma from a year ago.

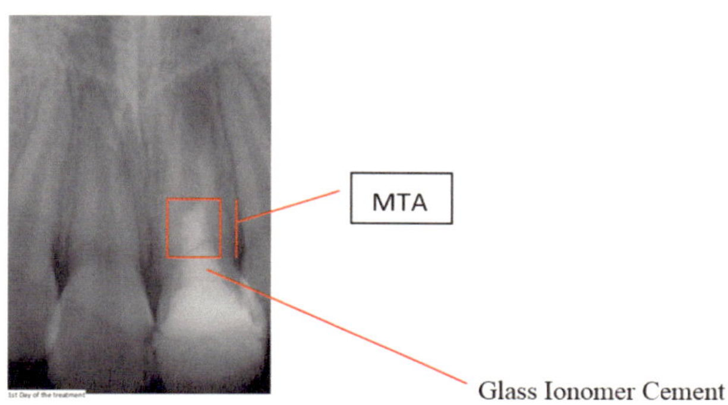

Figure 19.
First day of treatment: it is clearly seen that the root canal is very large, and the dentin walls are very thin.

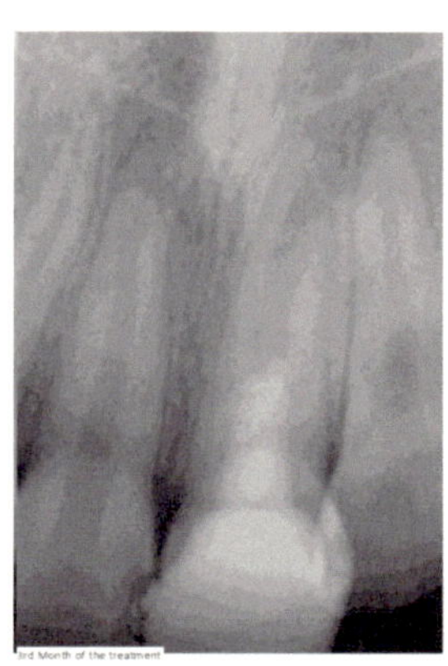

Figure 20.
Third month of the treatment: the lateral walls were thickened by the continued growth of dentin/hard tissue and the root length was increased.

If the treatment becomes success, in clinical and radiographical follow-ups, there should be no pain or swelling, apical radiolucency should be disappeared (usually observed 6–12 months after treatment), the root canal walls should be thickened (observed before the increase of the root length between 12 and 24 months), and the root length should be prolonged. Pulp should respond positively to vitality tests.

If there is no evidence of recovery, if the fistula does not disappear, and pain and swelling persist or no root growth is observed within 3 months, apexification with calcium hydroxide or MTA can be tried.

If pulp necrosis develops afterward, traditional endodontic treatment protocols should be performed [16, 18, 19, 25, 28, 38, 41–44, 46–49].

8.5 The advantages of revascularization treatment

Revascularization can be completed in a single session after the infection is controlled, and there is no need for repeated sessions as in the treatment of calcium hydroxide. This is very economical.

The greatest advantage is that it can regenerate the vitality of the tooth and maintain the root development.

The lateral walls are supported by the continuation of the dentin/hard tissue deposition, and the durability of the root is increased [16, 18, 19, 25, 28, 38, 41–44, 46–49] (**Figures 18–20**).

Author details

Asli Topaloglu Ak*, Didem Oner Ozdas, Sevgi Zorlu and Pinar Kiymet Karataban
Department of Pediatric Dentistry, Dentistry Faculty of Istanbul Aydin University, Istanbul, Turkey

*Address all correspondence to: asliak@aydin.edu.tr

References

[1] Marcenes W, Murray S. Social deprivation and traumatic dental injuries among 14-year-old schoolchildren in Newham, London. Dental Traumatology. 2001;**17**:17-21

[2] Oldin A, Lundgren J, Nilsson M, Norén JG, Robertson A. Traumatic dental injuries among children aged 0-17 years in the BITA study—A longitudinal Swedish multicenter study. Dental Traumatology. 2015;**31**:9-17

[3] Pattussi MP, Hardy R, Sheiham A. Neighbourhood social capital and dental injuries in Brazilian adolescents. American Journal of Public Health. 2006;**96**:1462-1468

[4] Petti S, Tarsitani G. Traumatic injuries to anterior teeth in Italian schoolchildren: Prevalence and risk factors. Endodontics & Dental Traumatology. 1996;**12**:294-297

[5] Rocha MJC, Cardoso M. Traumatized permanent teeth in Brazilian children assisted at the Federal University of Santa Catarina, Brazil. Dental Traumatology. 2001;**17**:245-249

[6] Rodd HD, Chesham DJ. Sports-related oral injury and mouthguard use among Sheffield school children. Community Dental Health. 1997;**14**:25-30

[7] Shulman JD, Peterson J. The association between incisor trauma and occlusal characteristics in individuals 8-50 years of age. Dental Traumatology. 2004;**20**:67-74

[8] Traebert J, Peres MA, Blank V, Böoell RD, Pietruza JA. Prevalence of traumatic dental injury and associated factors among 12-year-old school children in Florianópolis, Brazil. Dental Traumatology. 2003;**19**:15-18

[9] Andersson L, Andreasen JO. Important considerations for designing and reporting epidemiologic and clinical studies in dental traumatology. Dental Traumatology. 2011;**27**:269-274

[10] Andersson L, Kahnberg K-E, Oral PMA. Maxillofacial Surgery. Oxford: Wiley-Blackwell; 2010

[11] Andersson L. Epidemiology of traumatic dental injuries. Pediatric Dentistry. 2013;**35**(2):102-105

[12] Andreasen JO, Andreasen FM, Andersson L. Textbook and Color Atlas of Traumatic Injuries to the Teeth. 4th ed. Oxford: Blackwell Munksgaard; 2007

[13] Andreasen JO, Ravn JJ. Epidemiology of traumatic dental injuries to primary and permanent teeth in a Danish population sample. International Journal of Oral Surgery. 1972;**1**:235-239

[14] Chen YL, Tsai TP, See LC. Survey of incisor trauma in second grade students of Central Taiwan. Chang Gung Medical Journal. 1999;**22**:212-219

[15] July 2018. Available from: www.iadt-dentaltrauma.org (Accessed 20 July 2018)

[16] Banchs F, Trope M. Revascularization of immature permanent teeth with apical periodontitis: New treatment protocol? Journal of Endodontia. 2004;**30**(4):196-200

[17] Borsse'n E, Holm AK. Traumatic dental injuries in a cohort of 16-year-olds in northern Sweden. Endodontics & Dental Traumatology. 1997;**13**:276-280

[18] Chisini LA, Grazioli G, Francia A, San Martin AS, Demarco FF, Conde MCM. Revascularization versus apical barrier technique with mineral trioxide

aggregate plug: A systematic review. Giornale Italiano di Endodonzia. 2018;**32**(1):9-16

[19] Cotti E, Mereu M, Lusso D. Regenerative treatment of an immature, traumatized tooth with apical periodontitis: Report of a case. Journal of Endodontia. 2008;**34**:611-616

[20] Glendor U. Epidemiology of traumatic dental injuries: A 12 year review of the literature. Dental Traumatology. 2008;**24**:603-611

[21] American Association of Endodontists. Glossary of Endodontic Terms, 9th Edn: Chicago. http://www.nxtbook.com/nxtbooks/aae/endodonticglossary2016/index.php (Accessed 15 August 2018)

[22] Granville-Garcia AF, de Almeira Vieira IT, da Silva Siqueira MJP, et al. Traumatic dental injuries and associated factors among Brazilian preschool children aged 1-5 years. Acta Odontológica Latinoamericana. 2010;**23**:47-52

[23] Gronthos S, Brahim J, Li W, Fisher LW, Cherman N, Boyde A, et al. Stem cell properties of human dental pulp stem cells. Journal of Dental Research. 2002;**81**:531-535

[24] Eilert-Petersson E, Andersson L. S€orensen S. Traumatic oral vs. non-oral injuries. An epidemiological study during one year in a Swedish county. Swedish Dental Journal. 1997;**21**:55-68

[25] Giuliani V, Baccetti T, Pace R, Pagavino G. The use of MTA in teeth with necrotic pulps and open apices. Dental Traumatology. 2002;**18**:217-221

[26] Glendor U, Andersson L, Andreasen JO. Economic aspects of traumatic dental injuries. In: Andreasen JO, Andreasen FM, Andersson L, editors. Textbook and Color Atlas of Traumatic Injuries to the Teeth. 4th ed. © 1981, 1994 by Munksgaard, Copenhagen, Denmark © 2007 Blackwell Munksgaard A Blackwell Publishing Company

[27] Hamilton FA, Hill FJ, Holloway PJ. An investigation of dentoalveolar trauma and its treatment in an adolescent population. Part 1: The prevalence and incidence of injuries and the extent and adequacy of treatment received. British Dental Journal. 1997;**8**:182

[28] Hargreaves KM, Geisler T, Henry M, Wang Y. Regeneration potential of the young permanent tooth: What does the future hold? Pediatric Dentistry. 2008;**30**(3):253-260

[29] Hedegård B, Stålhane I. A study of traumatized permanent teeth in children aged 7-15 years. Part I. Swedish Dental Journal. 1973;**66**:431-450

[30] Holland TJ, O'Mullane DM, Whelton HP. Accidental damage to incisors amongst Irish adults. Endodontics & Dental Traumatology. 1994;**10**:191-194

[31] Dean JA. McDonald and Avery's Dentistry for the Child and Adolescent-E-Book. 10th ed. St. Louis, Missouri: Elsevier Health Sciences; 2015

[32] Kaste LM, Gift HC, Bhat M, Swango PA. Prevalence of incisor trauma in persons 6 to 50 years of age: United States, 1988-1991. Journal of Dental Research. 1996;**75**:696-705

[33] Marcenes W, Murray S. Changes in prevalence and treatment need for traumatic dental injuries among 14-year-old children in Newham, London: A deprived area. Community Dental Health. 2002;**19**:104-108

[34] Levin L, Friedlander LD, Geiger SB. Dental and oral trauma and mouthguard use during sports activities in Israel. Dental Traumatology. 2003;**19**:237-242

[35] Malikaew P, Watt RG, Sheiham A. Prevalence and factors associated with traumatic dental injuries (TDI) to anterior teeth of 11-13 year old Thai children. Community Dental Health. 2006;**23**:222-227

[36] Traumatic Dental Injuries AAE (Patient Education Brochure)

[37] July 2018. Available from: http://www.aapd.org/media/policies_guidelines/g_trauma.pdf (Accessed 20 July 2018)

[38] Namour M, Theys S. Pulp revascularization of immature permanent teeth: A review of the literature and a proposal of a new clinical protocol. The Scientific World Journal. 2014;**2014**:737503. DOI: 10.1155/2014/737503

[39] Tsukiboshi M. Treatment Planning for Traumatized Teeth. 2nd ed. Chicago: Quintessence Publ. Comp. Inc; 2012

[40] Koch G, Poulsen S, Espelid I, Haubek D. Pediatric Dentistry: A Clinical Approach. 3rd ed. Copenhagen, Denmark: John Wiley & Sons; 2017

[41] Vinchurkar S, Patil V. Outcomes of regenerative endodontic procedure In immature permanent teeth with necrotic pulps using different antimicrobial agents and/or Intracanal medicaments using different protocols: A systematic review. International Journal Of Scientific Research. 2018;**7**(3):37-43

[42] Garcia-Godoy F, Murray PE. Recommendations for using regenerative endodontic procedures in permanent immature traumatized teeth. Dental Traumatology. 2012;**28**(1):33-41

[43] Trope M. Regenerative potential of dental pulp. Pediatric Dentistry. 2008;**30**(3):206-210

[44] Theilade E. The microbiology of the necrotic pulp. In: Bergenholtz G, Horsted-Bindslev P, Reit C, editors. Textbook of Endodontology. 4th ed. Oxford: Blackwell, Munksgaard; 2007

[45] Reynolds K, Johnson JD, Cohenca N. Pulp revascularization of necrotic bilateral bicuspids using a modified novel technique to eliminate potential coronal discolouration: A case report. International Endodontic Journal. 2009;**42**(1):84-92

[46] Sato T, Ando-Kurihara N, Kota K, Iwaku M, Hoshino E. Sterilization of infected root-canal dentine by topical application of a mixture of ciprofloxacin, metronidazole and minocycline in situ. International Endodontic Journal. 1996;**29**:118-124

[47] American Association of Endodontists. AAE Clinical Considerations for a Regenerative Procedure [Internet]. Chicago: American Association of Endodontists; 2018. Available from: https://f3f142zs0k2w1kg84k5p9i1o-wpengine.netdna-ssl.com/specialty/wp-content/uploads/sites/2/2018/06/ConsiderationsForRegEndo_AsOfApril2018.pdf [Accessed: Jan 4, 2018]

[48] Regenerative Endodontics. Endodontics: Colleagues for Excellence. Chicago: American Association of Endodontists; 2013

[49] Yamauchi N, Yamauchi S, Nagaoka H, Dugan D, Zhong S, Lee SM, et al. Tissue engineering strategies for immature teeth with apical periodontitis. Journal of Endodontia. 2011;**37**:390-397

Section 5

Mandibular Fractures

Chapter 5

Evaluation and Management of Mandibular Fracture

Guhan Dergin, Yusuf Emes and Buket Aybar

Abstract

The mandibular bone is an important component of the facial bone, which has a unique role in digestive system, speech, and facial esthetics. For these important functions of mandibular bone, it is vital that surgeons should not only treat function but also consider the esthetics together. Mandibular fractures are among the most common traumatic injuries of the maxillofacial region. Even though treatment modalities are well established and being practiced for a long time, untreated and postoperative complications still decrease the patient's quality of life. This chapter aims to describe the cause, clinical presentations, diagnoses, and current treatment methods on the basis of resent literature.

Keywords: mandibular fracture, open reduction, rigid fixation, trauma

1. Introduction

The mandibular bone, which is an important anatomical and functional structure, constitutes the lower height and width of the facial skeleton. The mandible is a complex bony structure and has a vital anatomical articulation with other cranio-maxillofacial components. It has a fundamental function in digestive system and also plays an important role in speech and facial expression. The mandible is a v-shaped bone articulating with the temporal bone at the temporomandibular joint (TMJ). Mandibular bone has a horizontal and vertical portion.

The cartilaginous mandibular bone is a v-shaped bone articulating with the temporal bone at the temporomandibular joint (TMJ) [1]. Mandibular bone has a horizontal and vertical portion. The horizontal portion of mandible has two main structures, the basal and alveolar (tooth bearing) bones. Symphysis, parasymphysis, the body, and the alveolar bone compose the horizontal section of the mandible. The vertical mandible consists of the angle, ramus, condylar, and coronoid processes [2].

2. Brief historical overview

The first description of a mandibular fracture diagnosis and treatment goes back to the Egyptians in 1650 BC. Hippocrates described the reapproximation of fracture fragments and immobilization of the fractured mandible using circumdental wires and external bandaging.

Since then, many effective treatment methods and devices have been introduced to maxillofacial traumatology for the treatment of mandibular fracture including the facial bandage, extra oral fixation apparatus, intraoral acrylic, and metal splints, wires, arch bars, and stainless steel and titanium plate osteosynthesis. More recently resorbable screws and plates have been used for fracture management [3].

3. Etiology (epidemiology)

Mandible fractures have many different etiologies such as interpersonal violence, traffic accidents, gunshot wounds, sport accidents, work accidents, and falls [3]. The etiology of mandibular fractures varies from time to time, culture to culture. Students in different periods demonstrate differences in etiology depending on the age, demographic pattern of countries, and environmental conditions and social, socioeconomic, and cultural configurations. In developed countries, vehicle and sport accidents are main causes of mandibular fractures, while in developing countries and rural areas, inter personal violence, gunshot wounds, and falls in foregrounds [3–7].

4. Clinical and radiological assessment

4.1 Clinical

Complete history trauma should be obtained after cardiopulmonary and vital neurological functions of the patient are stabilized. Checking the airway by securing cervical spine is vital before assessment. Depending on the consciousness or neurologic status of the patient, history can be obtained from the patient or accompanying family members. Assessments including time, cause of trauma, pain, function of cranial nerves and altered sensation, visual changes, malocclusion, and general systemic conditions should be noted. Some mandibular fractures accompanying multiple injuries, as in traffic accidents, frequently require trauma team evaluation and consultation.

A neurologic examination is a vital point in the assessment of maxillofacial trauma. Functions of cranial nerves such as altered sensation, pupillary reflex, visual changes, and extraocular movements should be evaluated. Motor function of facial expression (nerve VII), symmetrical tongue movements, and mastication muscle (nerve V) should be checked. Sensation of the face should be also noted.

The mandible should be carefully evaluated by extraoral palpation. Mandibular contours such as ramus, lateral and inferior borders, and symphysis and parasymphysis area should be checked, and continuity of the mandibular bone should be noted. Movements of fragments can be evaluated by bidigital palpation. Ecchymosis and crepitation should be assessed. Check mandibular movements. Deviations and restriction of movements should be evaluated considering condylar trauma. Also the condylar head should be evaluated by palpation to check if it is in the articular fossa or not.

Mucosal laceration, oral bleeding, ecchymosis, and sublingual hematomas should be checked by the intraoral inspection. Rule out fresh oral bleeding in the sublingual space or bilateral symphysis fracture to secure airway, especially for anticoagulant drug users. Examination of the occlusion including loose, fractured, or missing teeth should be performed carefully.

4.2 Radiological

In most cases clinical examination cannot be sufficient to intensively evaluate the entire fractures lines, displaced small fragments, root fractures of teeth, and neighboring anatomical structures [8]. Plain films, OPTG, and computed tomography (CT) can provide additional data about the fracture for better evaluation of the patient. Periapical or occlusal radiographs are useful and practical imagining techniques for viewing specific areas of concern [9].

Although it is expensive, computed tomography (CT) is the most comprehensive imagining technique for evaluation of maxillofacial traumas. Detailed 0.5 mm thick slices provide excellent axial, coronal, and sagittal assessments of fracture lines, neighboring anatomical structures such as nerves. Also high velocity impaction traumas with multiple injuries require extensive stabilization of the patient. Additionally, 3D evaluations help to provide models for reconstruction and they are essential for proper approximations of fracture fragments with prepended titanium plates. Nowadays the use of cone-beam computed tomography (CBCT) in maxillofacial surgery has been providing less radiation and an accurate and reliable imagining alternative to conventional CT [10, 11].

Rarely, angiography and embolization can be used in the treatment of displaced TMJ fracture. Also MRI imagining can be helpful to evaluate soft tissue injuries such as TMJ disc.

4.3 Classification of mandibular fractures

Mandible fractures have a unique property within the maxillofacial traumas considering their history and treatment approach. The cornerstone of understanding the mandibular fractures is the classification of mandibular fractures. There are many fracture classifications in literature based on the type of fracture, cause of the fracture, reducibility, anatomic site, condition and inter-fragmental situation, and the presence of dentate or edentate segments. Some of these classifications are more widely accepted and used, and some of them are mostly seen in books but not used practically. Mandibular fractures are most commonly described as their anatomic location [3].

4.4 Fracture classifications based on anatomic site

1. Angle

2. Alveolar process

3. Body

4. Condyle

5. Coronoid

6. Ramus

7. Symphysis/parasymphysis

Fractures can be also classified as pathologic Fractures and traumatic fractures. Pathological fractures occur due to the failure of the bone which has lost its mechanical strength as a result of a pathological condition such as tumors, cysts, infections, etc. Traumatic fractures occur due to an impact which disrupts the continuity of the osseous tissue.

5. Biomechanics

The mandibular bone is exposed to many kinds of linear and angular forces underload such as compression and tension, shear, torsion, and bending [12]. External forces cause mandibular bone to undergo plastic and elastic deformation. On the other hand, muscles have some vertical and horizontal forces on fragments. These forces may cause displacement of fragments or may act as a stabilizer for fragments. The temporalis, masseter, and medial pterygoid muscle pull are responsible for vertical displacements of fragments. Horizontal displacements are mainly caused by lateral and medial pterygoid muscle pull. Some muscles have complex force on fragments such as mylohyoid, digastric, and geniohyoid which have a torsion effect on fragments.

Champy and co-workers described a zone of tension in the alveolar part of the mandible and a zone of compression on the lower border. This information allowed ideal lines for mandibular internal fixation to be identified along the physiological tension lines [3].

5.1 Muscle forces

Muscles have pull direction, and this pull effect may compress fragments to each other and prevent displacement. Fractures under the effect of these kinds of muscle pull vector are called favorable fractures.

On the other hand, some muscle pulls cause displacements of fragment. Fractures at these kinds of disadvantageous situations are called unfavorable

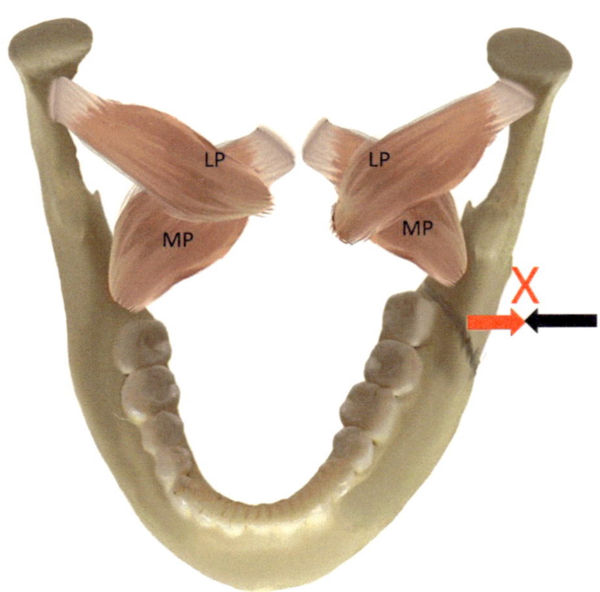

Figure 1.
Horizontally favorable fractures.

fractures. Favorable/unfavorable fracture concept is essential for mandibular fracture treatment decision which will be discussed later in this chapter.

Horizontally favorable fractures: reduced biomechanically by the masseter and temporalis muscle pull (**Figure 1**).

Horizontally unfavorable fractures: Displacement of fracture fragments increased or is provoked by the masseter and temporalis muscle pull (**Figure 2**).

Vertically favorable fractures: The pull vector of the pterygoid muscle promotes the reduction of the fracture segments (**Figure 3**).

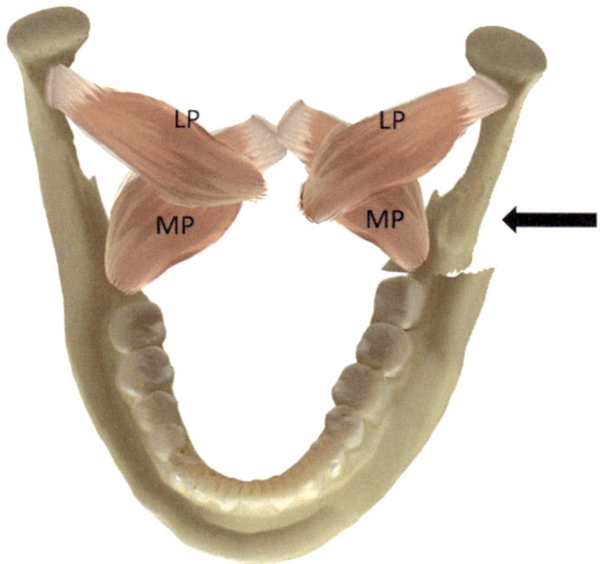

Figure 2.
Horizontally unfavorable fractures.

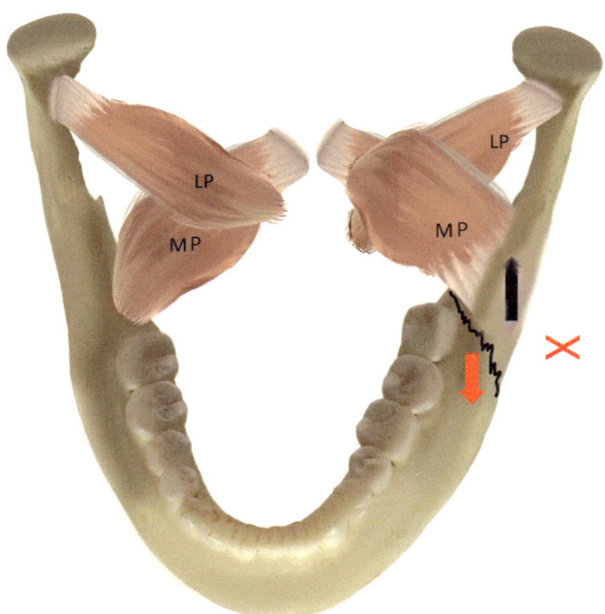

Figure 3.
Vertically favorable fractures.

Vertically unfavorable: The actions of the pterygoids tend to displace the fracture (**Figures 3 and 4**).

5.2 Tension and compression zones

Pulling force applied by muscles of oro-maxillofacial region creates zone of compression and tension within the mandible. The superior portion of the mandible is termed as the tension zone, and the inferior portion is termed as the compression zone (**Figure 5**). Champy's principle of osteosynthesis lines is based on these tension

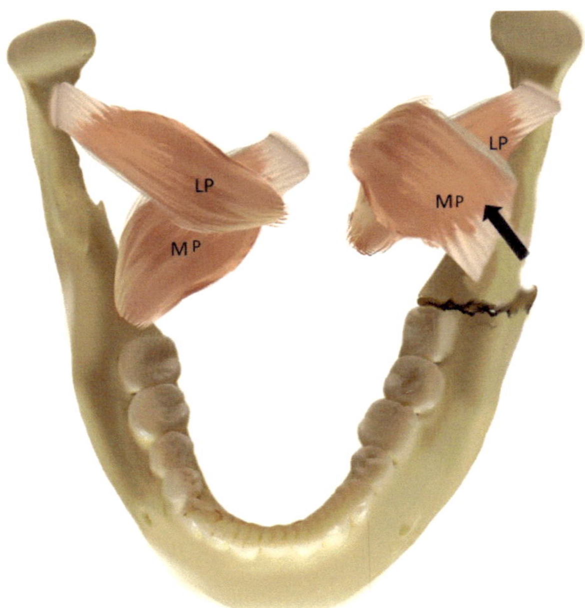

Figure 4.
Vertically unfavorable fractures.

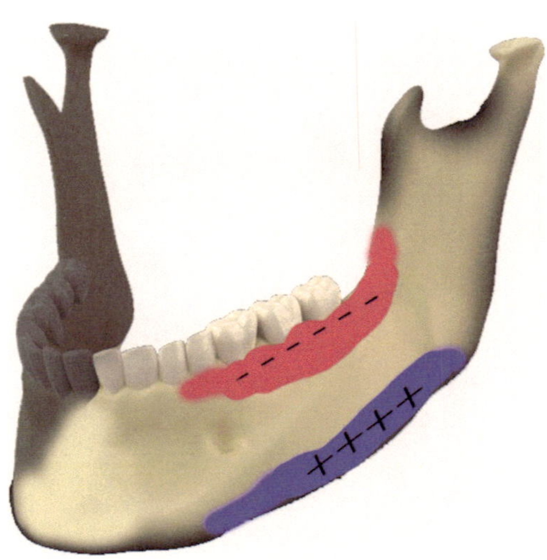

Figure 5.
Tension zone marked in red (−) and compression zones marked in blue (+).

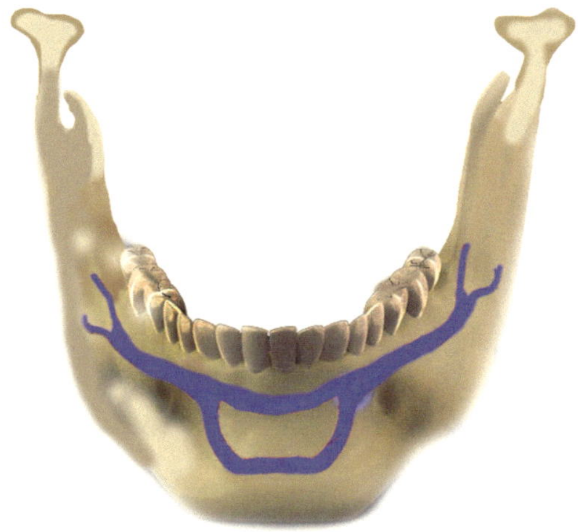

Figure 6.
Champy's principle of osteosynthesis lines.

and compressions zones which has been proven to be the guiding line to establish effective treatment for open reduction of mandibular facture (**Figure 6**) [3, 13].

6. Principle of mandibular fracture treatment

The trauma patient should first be provided with airway clearance. In a patient lying in the supine position, foreign bodies such as missed pieces of broken teeth and intraoral bleedings may create a danger of closing the airway. Although the blood in the mouth may be swallowed by the unconscious patient at first, it may cause vomiting as time passes. Breathing can be provided by pulling the mandible forward with a properly positioned cervical collar. It must be kept in mind that in patients with compound fractures, it may be difficult to position the lower jaw with the help of a cervical collar.

Antibiotics are preferred especially in open fractures and delayed healing. The patient should be given anti-inflammatory drugs, and if there are no clean wounds, the necessity of tetanus vaccine should be considered.

6.1 Prognosis of the teeth in the fracture line

Fractures of the fracture line, excessively displaced, and teeth which have their cement exposed, if they are not to be temporarily held in the mouth to maintain occlusion, must be extracted [14].

The teeth with apical infection and teeth with excessive periodontal defects, teeth with root fractures, and teeth that prevent the reduction of fracture segments should be extracted [15] (**Figure 7**).

6.2 Aim of fracture treatment

The purpose of fracture treatment is to return the mechanical strength of the fracture site to its healthy state and to achieve an improvement in the masticatory muscles' normal functions.

The first stage of treatment is to return the fracture parts to their normal anatomic position (reduction). The second stage is the fixation of the parts in their

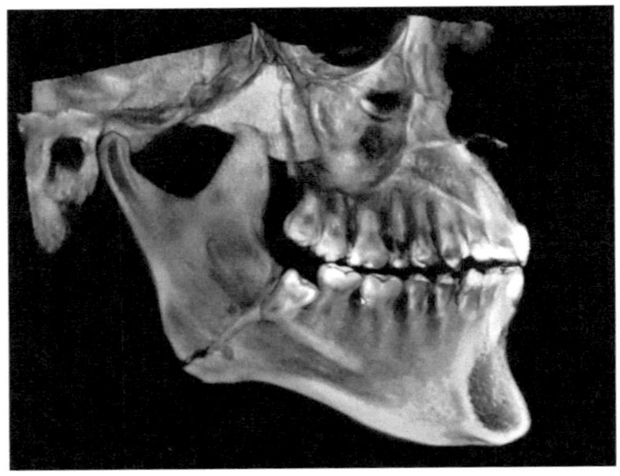

Figure 7.
Teeth that prevent the reduction of fracture segments.

normal anatomical position (fixation). If the history of the trauma does not exceed 8–10 days, the fixation of the fractures can be done manually. In order to control the pain, local anesthesia can be applied. Mobile dentoalveolar structures must be fixed using wires or similar methods [16].

6.3 Closed versus open treatment

Fractures of the mandible can be treated either with open method or closed method.

6.3.1 Closed reduction

Anatomically restoration of the fragments without visualization the fracture line is called closed reduction. In closed reduction both tooth-borne and bone-borne stabilization can be used to immobilize fracture to obtain correct maxilla-mandibular relation which is called intermaxillary fixation (IMF). Intermaxillary fixation (IMF) which is also called maxillomandibular fixation (MMF) is usually the basis of closed methods. Intermaxillary fixation is fixing the mandible and maxilla together when the teeth are occluded so that the patient cannot open his/her mouth for a certain period to allow secondary healing. The patient should be prescribed analgesics. One week of antibiotic use is required if there is an open fracture. The treatment continues until the hard callus is formed (4–6 weeks). Optimum bony union can be established in 4–6 weeks, but in complicated fractures, or compromised patients longer treatment periods can be required for healing. Closed method is still used today due to the advantage of elastic traction which helps successful repositioning of the fragments and its low cost. Arch bars, IVY loops, and intermaxillary fixation screws are all well-known appliances for closed reduction methods [17].

The use of vacuum-formed splints has also been recommended in the past for closed reduction.

In the closed methods, arch bars are often used with ligature wires. The wire is passed through the interdental gap. One end of the wire is passed under the arch bar, and the other end is passed over the arch bar. With a fine-tipped tool, the wire is placed under the cingulum of the tooth, and the wire is bent to secure the arch bar to the tooth.

Intermaxillary fixation screws are also used to obtain the occlusion in open reduction. However iatrogenic root injury is a major concern for this method. Also loosening of the screw and covering of the screw head with oral mucosa and screw fractures have been reported as complications regarding the use of IMF screws.

The most important disadvantage of closed therapy is the continuation of intermaxillary fixation for 4 weeks. This may lead to undernourishment of the patient and weight loss. Also the patient must be informed about oral hygiene due to difficulty in cleaning the teeth under IMF. Non-displaced favorable fractures and grossly comminuted fractures with soft tissue lost can be the candidate of closed reduction. Edentulous mandibular fractures are also controversial cases which mostly require periosteal blood supply. Some authors suggest closed reduction with gunning splints and circummandibular wires. On the other hand, some other authors claim that open reduction with minimum periosteal striping can be a good alternative for such cases [18].

6.3.2 Open reduction

Open reduction is preferred when closed treatment is not possible or has failed. In open reduction, there is a surgical approach to the fracture, and the fracture segments are repositioned to their anatomical positions. This stage is called reduction. This is followed by the fixation step. Fixation can be either rigid or semirigid in open reduction. Compression plates and bicortical screws are used in rigid fixation.

While this is a reliable method and allows the patient to quickly return to daily functions, this technique has some disadvantages [19].

Semirigid fixation is performed using mini-plates. These smaller plates are placed on the stress areas in the fracture area. It is thought that micromovements caused by semirigid fixation have a positive effect on the callus formation. Monocortical screws are used so that anatomical structures are preserved. It may be possible to perform even under local anesthesia and with an intraoral approach. Occasionally occlusion can be obtained using intermaxillary fixation and elasticity.

The patient is given a soft diet during semirigid fixation. It is not mandatory to remove the plates after healing [20].

6.3.2.1 Indications for closed reduction

- -No or little displacement.
- Little or no fracture mobility.
- Possibility of regaining pre-injury occlusion.
- The absence of infection.
- The patient's cooperation can be maintained and the follow-up is possible.
- Closed reduction can also be preferred in patients whom a surgical approach is not recommended, such as patients having fractures due to medicine-related osteonecrosis of the jaws.

6.3.2.2 Disadvantages of rigid fixation

- External approach may be required (requires skin incision and scar risks).
- The risk of damage to the alveolar is inferior and tooth roots.
- The need for a second surgical procedure to remove the plates.

6.3.2.3 Condyle fractures

When closed reduction is delayed in condyle fracture patients, open reduction may be required. The delaying of closed reduction causes muscles to spasm and prevent a successful repositioning of the fragments. Also medial pterygoid and temporalis muscles may get fibrotic when the treatment is delayed. As more time passes, the risk of ankylosis increases in the untreated condyle fracture patient.

When an open reduction of the condyle fracture is planned, usually and extraoral approach is required. The most common incision fort his procedure is the preauricular incision which directly leads to the temporomandibular joint. Another approach is the submandibular incision which does not involve the temporal mandibular joint directly.

Sometimes, to obtain reduction of the fragments, an intraoral incision at the sigmoid notch region may be used [21, 22].

6.3.2.4 Ramus fractures

Ramus fractures rarely require reduction. Chewing muscles adhering to the area effectively splint fractures. Elastic IMF is applied if occlusion is affected (**Figure 8**).

6.3.2.5 Angulus fractures

Triangular in shape, mandibular angle is the anatomic region between anterior border of masseter ligaments attachments and the most posterior superior attachment of masseter muscle. Angle fractures are anatomically unique regions that are developed laterally by the masseter and medially by medial pterygoid muscles which may stabilize the fracture in same situations. Vertical and horizontal fracture lines of this kind of fracture are essential fort the reduction of choice. Also the presence of unerupted third molars in this region is the weak point of this anatomical region. Unfavorable fractures of angle fracture may displace medially. Accompanying fractures such as condyle may alter the displacement of angle fractures.

Access to the site is provided through various incisions, and incisions are made along the external oblique line. The plates should be placed so that they will not be directly under the incision line. Sometimes a transbuccal approach using a trocar may be required. Extraoral approaches may also be rarely used for angulus comminuted or pathological fracture reduction with Risdon incision just 1 cm bellow the angulus. Open reduction or closed reduction both can be used for this kind of fractures considering the complexity, age, displacement, and accompanying fractures to the angulus fracture. In open reduction monocortical single plate at the superior border of angulus as Champy's method or bicortical two mini-plates

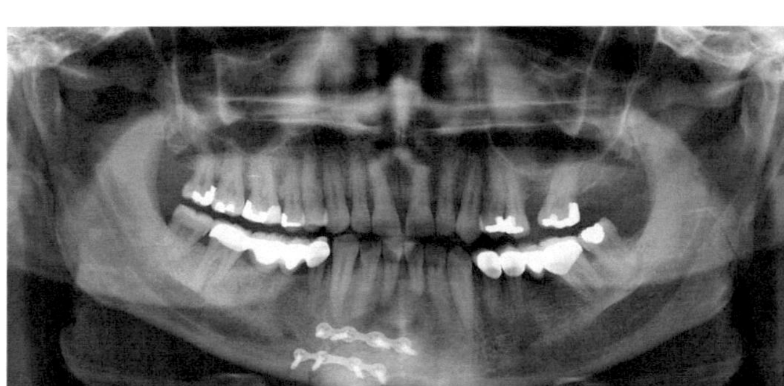

Figure 8.
Parasymphysis fractures accompanying ramus fractures, rarely require reduction.

can be selected as treatment method. Also the presence of uncontinuity defect or pathological fracture reconstruction plates should be consider fort the fracture managements. Load-sharing and load-bearing principles of fracture treatment must be the main guide as in all mandibular fractures [23] (**Figures 9** and **10**).

6.3.2.6. Symphysis/parasymphysis fractures

Considering the treatment plan, it should be noted that this region is under the influence of torsion forces. Open reduction, especially for unfavorable displaced fractures, is mostly preferred because of the easy access and complex forces upon symphysis/parasymphysis region. Also closed reduction can be used for favorable and non-displaced fracture. Champy's two-plate technique, one on tension and another on compression zone, is ideal for open reduction (**Figures 11–13**). Arch bar with one mini-plate at compression zone is also acceptable for fracture management. Anterior mandibular traumas should be evaluated very carefully.

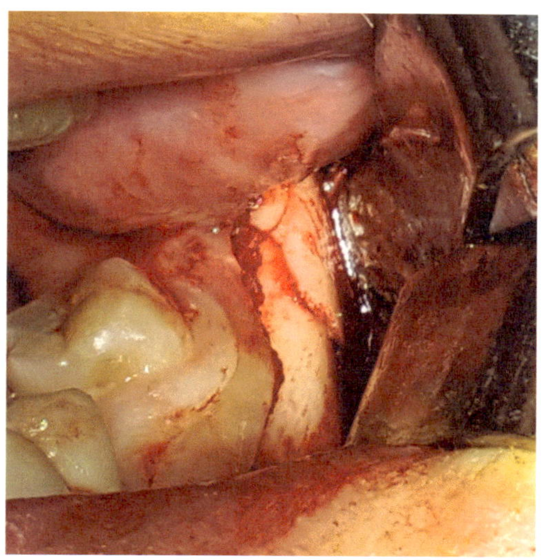

Figure 9.
Angulus fracture.

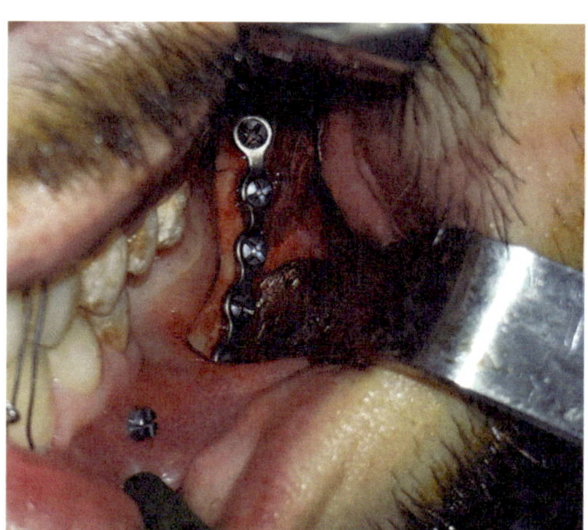

Figure 10.
Open reduction with monocortical single plate at the superior border of angulus as Champy's method.

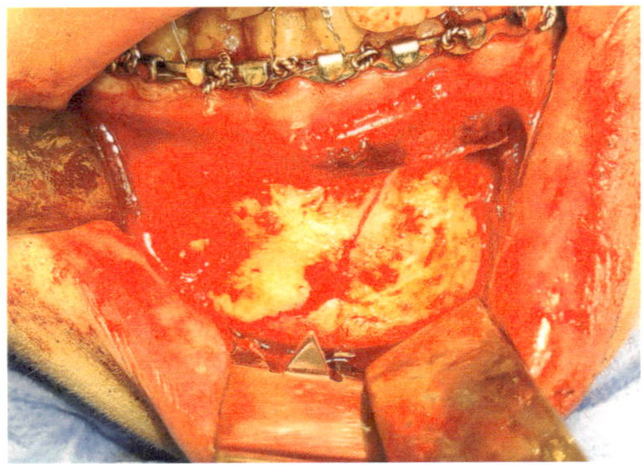

Figure 11.
Open reduction with monocortical with double plate, one at the superior border and the other at compression zone, as Champy's principle.

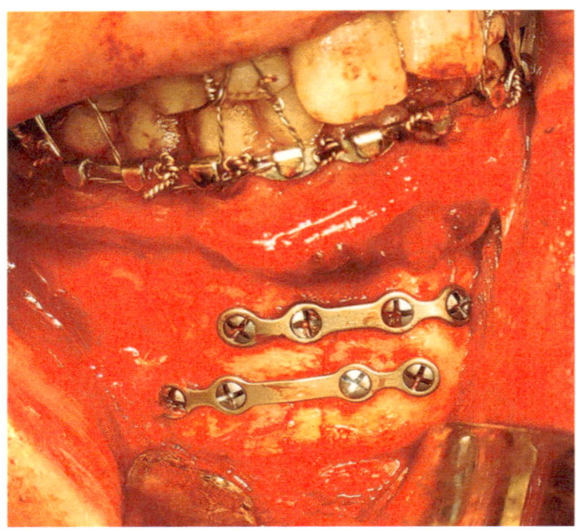

Figure 12.
Open reduction with mini plates.

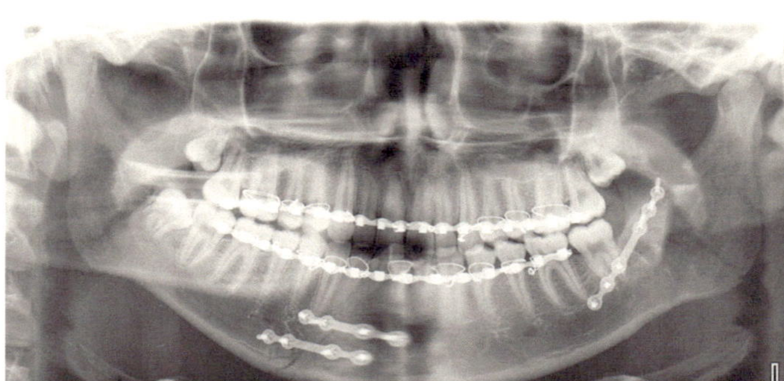

Figure 13.
Radiological view of open reduction of right parasymphysis fractures accompanying left angulus fracture.

Accompanying uni- or bilateral condyle fracture to symphysis/parasymphysis fractures is not rare.

Symphysis fractures can be treated either with closed or open reduction. Even though mini-plates are successful in the management of symphyseal fractures, some clinicians prefer lag screws for rigid fixation. Lag screws have the advantage of needing minimal time and a minimal intraoral incision similar to the incision for genioplasty, which has cosmetic advantages [24].

In the 1990s the use of 3D plates for the management of mandibular fractures has started to be recommended. Unlike compression plates and mini-plates, these 3D plates are placed on the week parts of the bone.

Even though not conclusive, recent studies show that 3D plates have better results in the condyle region with relatively poorer results in the body of the mandible, especially if the body is dentate.

6.3.2.7. Mandibular body fractures

Treatment principles of mandibular body fractures are based on Champy's line of osteosynthesis especially for simple fractures of the body. Intraoral access to this fracture is not difficult. One mini-plate at tension zone is sufficient for load-sharing fixation. Comminuted fractures may require additional mini-plates and screws. Also continuity defects such as pathological fractures need further load-bearing fixation systems such as reconplates. Mandibular continuity defects are defined as loss of the continuity of mandibular bone through a bone gap. Fractures close to mental foramen require additional care not to injure the mental nerve [17].

7. Timing of the surgical management

Just like other anatomical regions, all fractures involving the mandible should be treated as soon as possible. However, an immediate intervention is rarely applicable.

In patients who do not have airway problems and who do not have severe painful fractures, treatment can be delayed to the next day even though in cases of open fractures, the risk of infection increases as the time passes.

8. Complications

Infection is the most common complication within fracture management, especially in comminuted fractures and gunshots. Infection rates of authors vary between 0.4 and 32% [17, 25]. Postoperative infection increases the risks of the ununion and fibrous union of the fractures. Infection is not only the cause of the ununion or fibrous union of fractures, mobility and unstable fixation techniques also enhance ununion and fibrous unions in fractures. Fractures because of high-impact traumas, gunshot, or pathological fractures may cause hard and soft tissue lost which can result in esthetical and functional problems. In such cases extraoral surgical approaches may cause facial nerve damages. Inferior alveolar nerve injurious can be rarely seen in open reduction of parasymphysis and mandibular body fracture repairs. Hardware-related postoperative complications are hardware fails, screws and plate fractures, and tooth roots jeopardized by fixation screws.

9. Conclusion

Mandibula is one of the the main skeletal component of the face and their fractures are among the most common traumatic injuries of the maxillofacial region which jeopardize both esthetic and function patients. The occlusion, form, and function should be all considered in the managements of mandibular fractures.

Author details

Guhan Dergin[1]*, Yusuf Emes[2] and Buket Aybar[2]

1 Department of Oral and Maxillofacial Surgery, Faculty of Dentistry, Marmara University, Turkey

2 Department of Oral and Maxillofacial Surgery, Faculty of Dentistry, Istanbul University, Turkey

*Address all correspondence to: guhandergin@yahoo.com

References

[1] Stacey DH, Doyle JF, Mount DL, Snyder MC, Gutowski KA. Management of mandible fractures. Plastic and Reconstructive Surgery. 2006 Mar;**117**(3):48e-60e. DOI: 10.1097/01.prs.0000209392.85221.0b

[2] Abotaleb BM, Al-Moraissi E, Zhiqiang W, Ping C, Yongjie K, Alkebsi K, et al. A detailed analysis of mandibular fractures epidemiology, treatment and outcomes: A 5-year retrospective study, Gansu Province-China. Journal of Oral and Maxillofacial Surgery, Medicine, and Pathology. 2018;**30**:197-205. DOI: 10.1016/J.AJOMS.2017.12.001

[3] Fonseca RJ. Oral and Maxillofacial Surgery. Vol. 2. Saunders; 2017. pp. 146-172

[4] Lee K. Global trends in maxillofacial fractures. Craniomaxillofacial Trauma & Reconstruction. 2012 Dec;**5**(4): 213-222. DOI: 10.1055/s-0032-1322535

[5] Edwards TJ, David JD, Simpson DA, et al. Patterns of mandibular fractures in Adelaide, South Australia. Australian and New Zealand Journal of Surgery. 1994;**64**:307-311. DOI: 10.1111/j.1445-2197.1994.tb02216.x

[6] Ellis E, Moos KF, El-Attar A. Ten years of mandibular fractures: An analysis of 2,137 cases. Oral Medicine, Oral Pathology, Oral Surgery. 1985;**59**:120-129. DOI: 10.1016/0030-4220(85)90002-7

[7] Sakr K, Farag IA, Zeitoun IM. Review of 509 mandibular fractures treated at the University Hospital, Alexandria, Egypt. The British Journal of Oral & Maxillofacial Surgery. 2006;**44**:107-111. DOI: 10.1016/j.bjoms.2005.03.014

[8] Escott EJ, Branstetter BF. Incidence and characterization of unifocal mandible fractures on CT. American Journal of Neuroradiology. 2008;**29**:890-894. DOI: 10.3174/ajnr.A0973

[9] Romeo A, Pinto A, Cappabianca S, et al. Role of multidetector row computed tomography in the management of mandible traumatic lesions. Seminars in Ultrasound, CT, and MR. 2009;**30**:174-180. DOI: 10.1053/j.sult.2009.02.008

[10] Schuknecht B, Graetz K. Radiologic assessment of maxillofacial, mandibular, and skull base trauma. European Radiology. 2005 Mar;**15**(3):560-568. Epub 2005 Jan 21. DOI: 10.1007/s00330-004-2631-7

[11] Pickrell BB, Hollier LH. Evidence-based medicine: Mandible fractures. Plastic and Reconstructive Surgery. 2017 Jul;**140**(1):192e-200e. DOI: 10.1097/PRS.0000000000003469

[12] Draper ERC. Basic biomechanics. In: SPF H, ID MC, editors. Sciences Basic to Orthopaedics. WB Saunders Company Limited; 1998. Chapter 14. pp. 201-212

[13] Champy M, Loddé JP, Schmitt R, Jaeger JH, Muster D. Mandibular osteosynthesis by miniature screwed plates via a buccal approach. Journal of Maxillofacial Surgery. 1978;**6**(1):14e21. DOI: 10.1016/S0301-0503(78)80062-9

[14] Andreasen JO. Etiology and pathogenesis of traumatic dental injuries: A clinical study of 1298 cases. Scandinavian Journal of Dental Research. 1970;**78**:329-342. DOI: 10.1111/j.1600-0722.1970.tb02080.x

[15] Parameters of care. Clinical practice guidelines for oral and maxillofacial surgery (AAOMS ParCare 07); Version 4.0. Journal of Oral and Maxillofacial Surgery. 2007;238-24. (Suppl)

[16] Brandt MT, Haug RH. Open versus closed reduction of adult mandibular condyle fractures: A review of the literatüre regarding the evolution of current thoughts on management. Journal of Oral and Maxillofacial Surgery. 2003;**61**:1324-1332. DOI: 10.1016/S0278-2391(03)00735-3

[17] Omeje KU, Rana M, Adebola AR, Efunkoya AA, Olasoji HO, Purcz N, et al. Quality of life in treatment of mandibular fractures using closed reduction and maxillomandibular fixation in comparison with open reduction and internal fixation–A randomized prospective study. Journal of Cranio-Maxillo-Facial Surgery. 2014;**42**(8):1821-1826. DOI: 10.1016/j.jcms.2014.06.021

[18] Smith BR, Teenier TJ. Treatment of comminuted mandibular fractures by open reduction and rigid internal fixation. Journal of Oral and Maxillofacial Surgery. 1996;**54**:328-331

[19] Alpert B, Tiwana PS, Kushner GM. Management of comminuted fractures of the mandible. Oral and Maxillofacial Surgery Clinics of North America. 2009;**21**:185-192. DOI: 10.1016/j.coms.2008.12.002

[20] Chrcanovic BR. Open versus closed reduction: Comminuted mandibular fractures. Oral and Maxillofacial Surgery. 2013 Jun;**17**(2):95-104. Epub 2012 Jul 294. DOI: 10.1007/s10006-012-0349-2

[21] Zachariades N, Mezitis M, Mourouzis C, et al. Fractures of the mandibular condyle: A review of 466 cases. Literature review and reflections on treatment and proposals. Journal of Cranio-Maxillofacial Surgery. 2006;**34**:421-432. DOI: 10.1016/j.jcms.2006.07.854

[22] Khelemsky R, Moubayed SP, Buchbinder D. What is the evidence for open versus closed treatment of mandibular condylar fractures in adults? The Laryngoscope. 2016 Nov;**126**(11):2423-2425. DOI: 10.1002/lary.26076

[23] Ellis E, Walker LR. Treatment of mandibular angle fractures using one non-compression miniplate. Journal of Oral and Maxillofacial Surgery. 1996;**54**:864-867. DOI: 10.1016/S0278-2391(96)90538-8

[24] Kushner GM, Alpert B. Open reduction and internal fixation of acute mandibular fractures in adults. Facial Plastic Surgery. 1998;**14**(1):11-21. DOI: 10.1055/s-0028-1085298

[25] Koury M. Complications of mandibular fractures. In: Kaban LB, Pogrel AAH, Perrot D, editors. Complications in Oral and Maxillofacial Surgery. Philadelphia: WB Saunders; 1997. pp. 121-146

Section 6

Orthodontics

Chapter 6

Orthodontic Approach in Facial and Dental Trauma

Sanaz Sadry

Abstract

In this review, the prevalence of dental trauma, prevention and diagnosis of traumatic injuries, the effects of dental trauma in patients in need of orthodontic treatment, orthodontic intervention to dental traumatized teeth, and treatment options for poor anterior teeth due to trauma are discussed. Dental trauma is a condition that is frequently encountered in dentistry. When orthodontic treatment of traumatized teeth is planned, the orthodontist should be considered before orthodontic treatment and during orthodontic treatment. Prognosis is divided into two types as treatment options of bad anterior teeth, retaining the tooth in the mouth or pulling the tooth and restoration of the opening. The multidisciplinary teamwork and the role of the orthodontist in this team are important in order to achieve optimal results in the clinical intervention of these cases. Autotransplantation, orthodontic closure, or opening of the space are discussed when tooth extraction and toothless space restoration are required. It is very important to decide if orthodontic forces should be applied or not, and if orthodontic force is necessary, when should it be applied. Information on orthodontic forces applied to traumatized teeth was given in this chapter.

Keywords: orthodontic approach, dental trauma, tooth movement, autotransplantation, orthodontic space closure

1. Introduction

Dental trauma (traumatic dental injury) affects the teeth and soft and hard tissues around the oral cavity. According to research worldwide, dental trauma is often seen as a result of sporting activities, falls, traffic accidents, and fights and often requires emergency intervention [1, 2]. Because of the high rate of trauma in patients presenting with orthodontic treatment today, the orthodontist should plan how to perform dental movements in these patients and consider the long-term prognosis of these teeth before starting treatment. The orthodontists in the multidisciplinary team who intervenes in the trauma have a major role in obtaining optimal results in the traumatic tooth [3]. While interfering with dental trauma cases, treatment guidelines may not be applicable as standard for each patient. Each case should be evaluated and treated accordingly. General health of the patient, severity and type of the trauma, chronological and dental age of the patient, dental and anatomical development status, and whether the patient carries a device in the mouth during trauma are some of the factors determining the treatment. It is important to decide whether orthodontic force can be applied to dental traumatized teeth, and if it is to be applied, it will be applied after the trauma. Excessive amount of orthodontic force on dental teeth can cause undesirable effects such as root resorption [4, 5]. Patients with orthodontic attachments at the mouth during orthodontic treatment may also be exposed to dental trauma. When dental trauma occurs during orthodontic treatment, the path to be followed for treatment is based on clinical experience and individual case reports presented in the literature [3, 6, 7]. Dental injuries vary widely from simple enamel fractures to complicated fractures and often require complicated treatment of more than one type of injury. The knowledge and skills of the physician are very important in cases where such emergency treatment is required, and the first treatment is extremely important on prognosis [8].

2. Prevalence

Most of the dental trauma data available have been collected retrospectively from cross-sectional studies or from longitudinal studies of patient records. The prospective studies are based on subpopulations such as school children [9–12], children presenting to a pediatric dental service, or patients presenting to an accident and emergency department [13–15]. Permanent incisors of children that sustain damage by accident in the United Kingdom increases with age from 5% at age 8 to 11% by age 12, and injuries are more frequent in males than females [16–19]. Two comprehensive national studies conducted in the United States reported that one of six adolescents and one of four adults suffered traumatic dental injuries [20]. The majority of permanent tooth injuries occur in the age group of 6–15 and especially between the ages of 8 and 11 years. The upper teeth, especially the central incisors, are affected more by the lower teeth. This occurs more in boys than girls [21].

The researchers found that the injuries were mostly caused by traffic accidents, sports, and violence as a result of the incidents, and mostly due to falling in girls; they reported an uncomplicated crown fracture (55.4%), fracture (8.6%), complicated crown fracture (5.5%), luxation (4.3%), and avulsion (2.0%). Although the oral region of the human body constitutes 1% of the whole body, the statistics indicate that one fourth of the school age children and one third of the adults suffer from trauma [22].

3. Etiology

1. Human behavior: risk taking, problems experienced in relations with relatives, hyperactivity, and stress

2. Environmental factors: deprivation and overcrowding

3. Unconscious injuries: fall and crash, physical activities, traffic accidents, unsuitable teeth uses, and biting hard objects

4. Conscious injuries: physical exertion and iatrogenic procedures.

5. Predisposing factors: occlusal relationship, increased overjet amount, insufficient lip closure, history of previous trauma, and socioeconomic level [22].

The risk of trauma was found to increase as the amount of overjet increased. Incidence of trauma in the maxillary incisors was four times higher than the mandibular incisors. When the overbite was 0 mm, the risk of trauma in the mandibular incisors was the highest [23].

4. Classification

The WHO system was modified by Andreasen and Andreasen to further clarify the luxation and intrusion groups. This classification is as follows:

- Injuries involving hard tissues and pulp: Incomplete fracture of the crown, uncomplicated crown fracture, complicated crown fracture, and root fracture

- Supportive tissue injuries: Alveolar socket involvement (observed with intrusion and lateral luxation). Alveolar process fracture and maxilla mandibular fracture

- Gingiva or oral mucosa injuries: Gingiva or oral mucosa rupture, gingiva or oral mucosa injury, and abrasion of the gingiva or oral mucosa

The treatment plan for patients with traumatized tooth is evaluated in two parts as the prognosis of the traumatized tooth and the treatment of possible malocclusion [24].

5. Examination and diagnosis

Before an orthodontic treatment, a thorough anamnesis must be taken to determine whether the patient has suffered dental injuries. Before the examination, a comprehensive patient history is taken. The general health status of the patient, time of injury, and direct or indirect trauma are determined. In order to determine the state of the healing capacity of the tissues, whether the patient has been traumatized in the same area before, if any treatment has been performed in which the area, the tooth showing the damage in the support tissues or pulp, the sensitivity to spontaneous toothache, and hot-cold and sweet-sour foods are questioned. In the clinical examination, extraoral tissues, intraocular tissue, periodontal tissues, alveolar bone, and teeth are examined carefully. Abnormalities in the occlusion indicate a fracture in the alveolar and jaw. Sensitivity of the teeth during contact and whether the teeth are luxated are determined. According to the localization of the root fractures, there is luxation in the teeth. The mobility of the root fracture increases as the fracture line approaches the crown. Sensitivity to percussion refers to injuries in periodontal fibers. Thermal tests and vitalometer applications are used to determine the vitality of pulp in teeth injured due to trauma.

It is not always possible for the patient to remember whether he has had a dental injury, so that the patient should be evaluated clinically and radiographically prior to the treatment, and this evaluation should include the following:

The tooth should be checked for coloration and recorded. Crown yellow colorations, pulp canal obliteration; dark coloring may be a sign of pulpal hemorrhage or necrosis. It should be examined whether there is mobility in horizontal and vertical direction. With palpation, the apical area of the teeth should be checked for sensitivity. Percussion should be examined. In percussion, metallic sounds may be a sign of ankylosis, and blunt sounds may be a sign of root fracture. Thermal and electrical pulp tests and pulp response should be considered. Thermal tests were used to determine the neurovascular support of the traumatic tooth pulp; electrical pulp test plays an important role in determining the pulp necrosis of the tooth.

Radiographs are an important factor in the diagnosis of traumatic dental injuries. Depending on the type of malposition (e.g., lateral luxation) and the type of fracture (specimen, root fracture), it is important to take periapical film from various angles to perform an accurate examination.

Unexpectedly developing dental trauma may affect the oral function and psychology of the patient. It is necessary to eliminate the negative effects of pain and trauma on the teeth and periodontal tissues as soon as possible after dental trauma occurs in individuals receiving fixed orthodontic treatment. Regardless of the stage of fixed orthodontic treatment, dental trauma during treatment disrupts the routine functioning of active orthodontic treatment. The first emergency intervention in the trauma area is relieving of the pain, and the orthodontic force is rapidly removed from the teeth in the trauma area. Then, according to the severity of dental trauma, treatment is carried out with an individual approach that includes multidisciplinary treatment methods [20].

Brin et al. reported that increased overjet and insufficient lip closure were the greatest risk factors for dental trauma and that early orthodontic treatment to reduce overjet would reduce the risk of dental trauma. The use of mouthguard in individuals interested in contact sports is also an application that reduces the risk of dental injury [23, 24]. Bauss et al. reported different treatment approaches according to the type of dental trauma in patients with dental trauma during orthodontic treatment [7].

6. Treatment sequence and timing

Orthodontic treatment should usually be initiated during mixed dentition. When trauma occurs at an early age, the treatment will be shorter and less complicated, given the age, dental and skeletal development, and maturity of the patient [20].

7. Observation periods before orthodontic treatment

7.1 Crown and crown-root fractures

If crowns and crown-root fractures without pulp are treated appropriately, their prognosis is good. Before the orthodontic treatment, the 3-month observation period is sufficient. Crown and crown-root fractures containing the pulp can be treated orthodontically after partial pulpectomy and hard tissue barrier formation. Hard tissue barrier is observed radiographically 3 months after treatment [20].

This type of fracture includes enamel, dentin, and cement. Pulp may or may not be exposed. As a result of the traumatic forces that come out of the teeth, crown-root fractures are frequently encountered [25]. It has been reported that vertical crown-root fractures should be extracted. In diagonal crown-root fractures, the broken tooth must be orthodontically extruded to expose the subgingival fracture line [26]. The distance of healthy gingival tissue on the alveolar bone is defined as the biological width. This width is ideally considered to be equal to the sum of the connective tissue attachment (1 mm) to the sum of the epithelial attachment (1 mm). The extraction of the fractured tooth by obtaining the biological width is important for the ideal restoration of the tooth [25].

7.2 Luxated teeth

Clinical experiences showed that light injuries such as confusion and subluxation require at least a 3-month observation period. The need for endodontic treatment usually arises after moderate to severe limb injuries. Radiographic improvement revealed that orthodontic treatment should be postponed until it is out.

7.3 Endodontically treated teeth

Wickwire and colleagues compared root resorption of endodontically treated teeth with vital teeth after orthodontic treatment, and more root resorption was found in devital teeth [27]. Mirabella and Arthun suggested that endodontic application is a protective treatment and that root canal-filled teeth are resorbed for unknown reasons [28]. Hunter and colleagues in their study showed no difference between the vitality of vital and devital teeth root resorption after orthodontic treatment [29]. Hamilton and Gutman stated that if the root canal filling is properly shaped three dimensionally and cleaned, minimal resorption will be seen during the movement of orthodontic teeth [28].

7.4 Root canal calcified teeth

Calcification of the root canal is usually seen after autotransplantation of immature teeth, and these teeth can be moved in a limited manner. However, closely monitoring the root canal calcified teeth during orthodontic treatment is extremely important [20].

8. Special treatment principles in various trauma types

It is essential that radiographic examination is performed before starting orthodontic treatment, even in light injuries such as uncomplicated crown fracture. If the vitality of pulp is suspected, it is recommended to undergo a 3-month observation period before orthodontic treatment [20].

- Crown-root extrusion and cervical root fracture: This type of fracture includes enamel, dentin, and cement. Pulp may or may not be exposed. As a result of the traumatic forces that come out of the teeth, crown-root fractures are frequently encountered [30]. It has been reported that vertical crown-root fractures should be extracted. In diagonal crown-root fractures, the broken tooth must be orthodontically extruded to expose the subgingival fracture line [26]. The distance of healthy gingival tissue on the alveolar bone is defined as the biological width. This width is ideally considered to be equal to the sum of the connective tissue attachment (1 mm) and to the sum of the epithelial attachment (1 mm). The extraction of the broken tooth by obtaining the biological width is important for the ideal restoration of the tooth [30]. In crown-cervical or cervical root fractures, it may be necessary to orthodontically extrude the fractured root piece during restoration of the tooth. The fast extrusion technique has been developed to save these teeth. A hook is placed in the root canal with this technique, and the root is extruded in the axial direction [31]. Relapse may occur after orthodontic extrusion. Fibrotomy should be performed at least 3–4 weeks before the retention period to avoid relapse [32].

- Slow orthodontic extrusion: It is the extraction of the tooth with slow forces (20–30 gr). Biodiversity cannot be achieved by orthodontic extrusion only, because the movement of the teeth formed by orthodontic extrusion follows the gingiva and the alveolar bone. Orthodontic extrusion takes 4–5 months and then 12 weeks of retention. After orthodontic movement, periodontal surgery is needed to reshape the gingiva. Periodontal fibers can be cut to prevent recurrence (fiberotomy), and prosthesis can be applied 2–3 months later [30].

- Fast orthodontic extrusion: Under normal conditions, bone and gingival movement is performed by lightweight extrusive forces. When stronger pulling forces (> 50gr) are applied, rapid movement will exceed the physiological capacity of the tissues, and the movement in the support tissues is very low. After rapid extrusion is performed, a retention phase is required to adapt the periodontium to the new position of the tooth and allow the bone to be reshaped. The researchers reported that radiographs and histological analyzes revealed rare resorption in the root after rapid orthodontic extrusion [33].

- Root fractures: Dentin is broken into cement and pulp. Root fracture and luxation injuries can occur simultaneously; attention should be paid to root fractures. Post-traumatic root fractures are not frequently seen, and the incidence of post-traumatic root fractures in continuous teeth ranges from 0.5 to 7%. Horizontal root fractures are usually seen in the middle 1/3 of the root, followed by apical and coronal in the remaining 2/3 parts. Horizontal fractures are frequently seen in maxillary anterior teeth and in men aged 11–20 years. In general, root fractures have completed the continuation of the apex, and the teeth are affected. Simple fractures away from the cervical line have better prognosis [34]. In cases close to the cervical line, the fracture fragment can be excised with rapid extrusion, and crown restoration is possible [35]. If the granulation tissue and the coronal fragment are found to have necrosis among the fragments, endodontic treatment should be performed on the coronal fragment before orthodontic treatment. Following a successful canal treatment, the healing of the fracture line is caused by connective tissue. A 2-year observation period is recommended prior to orthodontic movement in teeth with root fracture, but this period can be reduced to 1 year if there is no complication [36].

Observation period prior to orthodontic treatment of the teeth with root fracture is determined as 2 years. Clinical experience has shown that most complications, such as pulp necrosis, occur 1 year after trauma. If no complication occurs, the observation period may be shortened. There are two types of treatment options, orthodontic or surgical extrusion, in teeth with complicated crown-root or cervical root fracture [20]. The orthodontic success of teeth with root fractures depends on the localization of the fracture and the type of healing. Radiographic and histological examinations showed that different types of healing are seen after root fractures: (1) Recovery with calcified tissues, (2) connective healing, and (3) improvement of bone growth between fractures. Healing with calcified tissues is the healing of the fracture with dentin and cement. Full interlocking of the fracture may not be completed, but the fracture has been combined. The orthodontic movement of the teeth with a hard tissue callus and a fractured root fracture can occur without the fracture line. The fracture margins are covered with cement and periodontal ligaments in the healing of the intervening tissues. Orthodontic movement of teeth with root fractures and broken pieces is separated from the connective tissue to move away from each other. In the orthodontic treatment plan of fractured teeth root with intervening connective tissues, the tooth should be seen as a short-rooted. This means that the teeth broken from apical one third have sufficient periodontal support for orthodontic tooth movement [37].

- Luxated teeth: In clinical examinations, it was found that if there was no resorption in the luxated teeth, it showed the same prognosis with non-traumatized teeth [38].

- Avulse teeth: In order to achieve a complete improvement in the avulsion injuries that occur in permanent teeth, the tooth must be inserted into the socket as soon as possible. Storing the avulsed tooth in milk for more than 60 minutes or 30 minutes dry causes ankylosis in the tooth after reimplantation [38, 39]. Orthodontic movement of the tooth is not recommended until after the reimplantation periodontal recovery is complete (6 months). It should be emphasized that the tooth may be ankylosis if orthodontic force is not performed as expected [3]. Replantation is considered primarily when the avulsed tooth is intact. Replantation is the insertion of the avulsed tooth into the alveoli with acute trauma. The loss of the permanent tooth after trauma is a condition that requires an orthodontic treatment plan. The main question is whether the cavity will be preserved for dental autotransplantation, implant placement, or bridge. Autotransplantation can be performed with both mature and immature teeth. However, in most cases with autotransplantation, the best prognosis is observed if the 3/4 of the tooth germ is formed or if the entire root is formed, but the apex is open. At this stage, the pulp maintains its vitality and continues its root development. Transplanted teeth lose only a small portion of the root length [21]. Bone-supported implants have been widely used instead of lost anterior teeth in recent years. Implants are fixated within the jaw and do not erupt during dental and alveolar development. For this reason, growth and development must be completed before implant placement [20].

- Space closure: Space formed of loss maxillary lateral incisors can be closed by positioning the maxillary canine in the lateral cutting region. Rather than the tooth that has been lost, rather than a prosthetic lateral tooth, the closure of the lateral tooth leads to more esthetic results periodontally. Canines are bled, to achieve more esthetic results. The length of the clinical crown can be changed through gingivectomy [40]. Following the orthodontic closure of the lost central tooth, if the shifted teeth are decided to be reshaped, the lateral tooth intrusion and the canine tooth are extruded to obtain the gingival contour of the central and lateral teeth [41]. In cases where the maxillary central teeth are lost, it is a complex condition where the lateral tooth is replaced by the mesial movement of the central tooth. The space is not fully closed, which poses risk. In cases where laterals are replacing the centrals, the lateral cutter should be raised in the mesiodistal direction, and the buccal root torque is required [42]. Extrusion of the canine tooth and intrusion of premolar teeth are performed in order to obtain the optimum gingival marginal contour of the anterior teeth. Lateral root torque is applied to the canine tooth and canine root torque to the repositioned premolar. Canine tooth is worn as composite or porcelain (porcelain veneers are more suitable and preferable) and restored to give it lateral form. The width of the canine tooth is reduced to provide optimal esthetic and functional occlusion by increasing the length and width of the first premolar teeth that are extruded and mesialized by composite restorations. The canine tooth with a more yellow color is bleached after its mesialization to the lateral tooth position [41].

In cases where the incisors are lost, the esthetic and functional results cannot be obtained by closing the space, and the completion of jaw growth should be expected. In this case, space should be maintained, and set-up models should be studied for different alternatives of tooth positions [43].

- Maintaining the space: The space can be maintained if it is not suitable. In patients with normal occlusion and dysesthesia with poorly aligned normal occlusion if more than one incisor is lost in the same arch, in class II division or class III patients who have lost one tooth in the upper jaw, there is a large discrepancy between the crowns of the central and lateral incisors and the space may be maintained in patients with lip deficiency [44]. Various space maintainers can be used to protect the space. The best option is to use the traumatized tooth as space maintainer when the prognosis is poor. But teeth should be checked. In case of ankylosing, it should be extracted without a severe infraocclusion [45].

- Opening of the space with orthodontic treatment: In their study, Kokich and Crabill applied an orthodontic site development technique to a 7-year-old patient who lost the central tooth due to avulsion. The researchers reported that the ongoing teeth would move massively instead of rolling over to the space and would carry the alveolar bone here. The neighboring teeth are allowed to move in the toothless space by applying a space maintainer until the tooth is complete. Since there was no stenosis in the patient, it was decided to reopen the toothless cavity, which was closed after the teeth, and place the implant. This technique is called "orthodontic site development." When the teeth are taken back to their original place, the missing tooth's cavity is filled with bone. With orthodontic site development, researchers have reported that bone does not undergo any resorption or contraction over time, thus providing a suitable site for implant placement [46].

- Autotransplantation: 43 years ago, Slagsvold and Bjercke developed a new method by transplanting partially formed teeth. In these teeth, endodontic treatment is usually not required after application. Most traumatic injuries are between 7 and 10 years of age, which makes it possible for autotransplantation of developing premolar. Dental autotransplantation has been reported to be a highly successful technique. Pediatric patients with orthodontic tooth extraction are suitable for autotransplantation [47]. Due to root anatomy, mandibular premolar teeth are preferred for this procedure. The most appropriate time for transplantation is when the 2/3 part of the root of the tooth is formed and has a larger apical opening of 1 mm. One hundred eighteen unfinished teeth were examined for 1–13 years, and in this period, 96% of the pulp regeneration rate was observed in the transplantation process [41]. Vilhjalmsson et al. [48] reported their success rate in autotransplantation as 80.5% in 2011. As the root growth of the tooth continues and normal periodontal ligament formation is observed, these teeth can be moved orthodontically without being different from the other teeth. It is recommended that the tooth be observed for 3–4 months before orthodontic movement [48].

- Crown and root malformations: Malformations of permanent teeth due to traumatic injuries sometimes cause permanent teeth to remain buried. If the root development of the tooth is sufficient, the tooth can be placed in the appropriate position by means of surgery and orthodontics [49].

- Intrusive teeth: In intrusion injuries, the tooth is displaced in the apical direction. Intrusion injuries are a type of trauma that is frequently encountered. Intrusion injuries lead to serious damage to the tooth, periodontium, and pulp. Ankylosis, pulp necrosis, and pulp calcification are among the most common adverse effects of traumatic intrusion. Special attention should be paid to these teeth during orthodontic treatment [30]. In severe intrusion injuries, periodontal ligament regeneration may occur, but a rapid progressive replacement resorption, marginal bone loss, inflammatory root resorption, ankylosis, and pulp necrosis may occur in less severe intrusion injuries [3].

The incidence of replacement resorption in intrusive cutters varies between 5 and 31%. The relationship between the severity of the intrusion and the type of root resorption was examined, and a significantly higher rate of replacement resorption was seen in the severely intrusive apex closed teeth [33].

Treatment: In the case of closed and severely intramedullary apex closed teeth, the tooth should be immediately placed in the previous alveolar position (early orthodontic extrusion) to allow the extirpation of non-vital pulp and to prevent the formation of inflammatory resorption. Since active surgery or orthodontic extrusion will cause a secondary trauma in the periodontal ligament, the teeth should be spontaneously re-erupted in individuals under 17 years of age who have suffered low and moderate trauma [39]. In 2 weeks, active extrusion may be considered if no movement occurs in the tooth. A serious intrusion force may compress the tooth in alveolus, thus the tooth can be lightly luxated prior to orthodontic extrusion [3].

Early orthodontic extrusion: For orthodontic extrusion of 1–2 teeth that have been intrinsic, extrusion force may be applied by using a movable apparatus and vertical elasticities between the teeth attached to the tooth. With this application, the reactive forces are aimed to be absorbed by the palatal mucosa under the acrylic instead of the adjacent teeth [50]. It is important to avoid anchoring from the neighboring teeth as much as possible in the treatment of a tooth affected by the intrusion. The use of conventional brackets and wire methods is not suitable in such cases, since the extent of the trauma that affected these teeth is unknown [50].

Success rate: early orthodontic extrusion prevents ankylosis [51].

- Immature teeth: If the intrusion and root end are not closed and the intrusion is too severe, it can be left to eruption or can be opened slightly by finger pressure. An orthodontic extrusion force is required if the intrusion is too severe or if the tooth does not start within 2–4 weeks [44].

- Replanted teeth: Most of the root resorption after replantation occurred within 1 year after the trauma. During this time, if there is no complication, the replanted tooth can be moved. Replanted and intrusive teeth show good prognosis in early recovery in 5 or 10 years after trauma and slow resorption can be seen [52].

- Ankylosis: In the adolescent growth phase, ankylosis causes the formation of an infraocclusion in the tooth. A metallic sound is detected in the ankylosis percussion by the absence of periodontal cavity. A clinically ankylosing tooth cannot be moved with orthodontic forces. Surgical luxation of the ankylosing tooth and leaving it for eruption or orthodontically extruding it is a successful method. In this technique, surgical luxation and ankylosing area are aimed to create connective tissue attachment and to move the tooth orthodontically [53]. Recently, good results have been reported in the case reports that the tooth was moved within a few weeks with the alveolar osteotomy and distraction osteogenesis of the ankylosing tooth [54–56]. Replanted avulse teeth often suffer from ankylosis. The root of the replanted tooth is gradually resorbed and replaced by bone. Ankylosis tooth growth in the developmental period does not follow the development of occlusion. In this phase, the tooth should be pulled, or the root should be left as space maintainer until it is resorbed [57]. When the alveolar growth is about to be completed, distraction osteogenesis and surgical block osteotomy can be performed to bring the tooth to the appropriate vertical position on the dental arch. The purpose of this method is to make the bone level suitable to facilitate subsequent prosthetic procedures. During this period, it should not be forgotten that the process of ankylosis continues [58, 59]. The progression of the infarction varies from individual to individual, depending on age, growth rate, and growth direction of the jaws. If the patient has a growth model, the infraposition is more severe. Severe infraposition, especially ankylosis with rapid alveolar growth, occurs if it occurs between the ages of 10 and 12. In such cases, the ankylosing tooth should be removed after 2 to 3 weeks following diagnosis [45].

- Extraction of ankylosing incisors: Decoronation technique has been developed to prevent bone loss in the extraction of ankylosing teeth. The crown of the ankylosing tooth is removed, and the stem is left in the alveoli. In children, a new marginal bone is formed to resorb the coronal root. Thus, the height of the alveolar bone increases vertically and is also preserved faciolingually [60].

9. The effect of orthodontic tooth movements on traumatized teeth

- Pulp vitality: In a study, Brin et al. stated that, in traumatic teeth, there was mostly no response to vitality tests following orthodontic treatment. Since there are few studies on this subject, it is not yet clear whether orthodontic dental movements increase the risk of pulp necrosis in traumatic teeth [61].

- Root resorption: If 20% of the root surface is affected by ankylosis, a metallic sound can be detected in percussion [38]. This is the first indication that ankylosis has begun to occur. Ankylosis usually begins to form on the buccal and palatal surfaces in the first stage, so it cannot be observed in conventional radiographs for up to 1 year. Following an injury, a 4–5-month observation period was recommended before any orthodontic force was applied [62]. Linge et al. reported that after orthodontic treatment, 1.07 mm resorption was observed in trauma teeth and 0.64 mm in unstressed teeth [62]. In patients who had trauma and root resorption, periapical radiographs should be taken 6–9 months after starting orthodontic treatment. If minor root resorption is seen and if it is decided to continue treatment, a radiograph should be taken again after 3 months, and the prognosis of resorption should be examined. If severe root resorption is observed, treatment should be ceased for 3 months. In maxillary incisor teeth with severe root resorption, permanent tooth mobility has been reported in cases where root length is less than 9 mm or equal to 9 mm [64, 65].

9.1 Prognosis

In mild to moderate luxation injuries (such as confusion or subluxation) of the teeth, if the orthodontic treatment is performed carefully, the risk of root resorption is reduced. After severe luxation (extrusion, lateral luxation, intrusion, and replantation), it is more dangerous to move the tooth. Orthodontic treatment is important to assess the risk of root resorption 6 months after onset. If progressive resorption is observed at this stage, treatment may be interrupted for 3 months to reduce the risk of severe resorption [66].

In conclusion, the prognosis of the whole treatment can be summarized as follows;

1. The prognosis of the traumatized tooth is good, and the prognosis of malocclusion is good: Treatment procedures for malocclusion are the same as untreated teeth the treatment procedures [20].

2. Good prognosis of traumatic tooth but poor prognosis of malocclusion: Orthodontic treatment is complex. It requires a long treatment period, and there are serious anchorage problems. In order not to overload the traumatized tooth, sometimes limited therapeutic purposes should be considered [20].

3. Poor prognosis of traumatic tooth but good prognosis of malocclusion: Traumatic tooth must be extracted but may be left as a space maintainer until the start of orthodontic treatment. The prognosis of orthodontic treatment is good, and optimal results are obtained [67].

4. Malignancy of the traumatized tooth is poor, and the prognosis of malocclusion is poor: Traumatic tooth must be extracted but can sometimes be left as space maintainer. Depending on the patient's age, the treatment options may include the use of prosthesis, implant, or the autotransplantation of premolar teeth [68, 69]. Orthognathic treatments may also be a treatment option [20].

9.2 Retention

During treatment, closure or preservation of the space is decided according to the retention period. Retention plan can be divided into three groups: group with limited retention and partial permanent retention. The need for retention of patients who are traumatically injured and undergoing orthodontic treatment depends on many factors. The most important ones [20] are the elimination of the cause of malocclusion, appropriate occlusion, reconstruction and reorganization of soft tissues and bone around placed teeth, and correcting skeletal deviations during growth development period. The need for retention is limited if these goals are achieved.

10. Result

Dental injuries are considered an emergency in dentistry. Increased overjet reduction and the use of mouthguard are protective applications that reduce the risk of dental trauma. The knowledge of the physician is of paramount importance in cases of dental trauma that require urgent treatment, and the first treatment is extremely important on prognosis. In trauma cases, the prognosis of traumatized tooth with existing malocclusion should be evaluated. After the treatment of traumatized teeth, the teeth should be evaluated clinically and radiographically at the end of the observation period required for orthodontic treatment. Dental trauma is generally seen in individuals who continue to grow and develop, and orthodontic treatment, which is a conservative method in the treatment of traumatized teeth, is an ideal treatment option that meets the esthetic and functional needs of patients.

Author details

Sanaz Sadry
Department of Orthodontics, Dentistry Faculty of Istanbul Aydin University, Istanbul, Turkey

*Address all correspondence to: sanazsadry@aydin.edu.tr

References

[1] Glendor U. Epidemiology of traumatic dental injuries a 12 year review of the literature. Dental Traumatology. 2008;**24**:603-611

[2] Lam R. Epidemiology and outcomes of traumatic dental injuries: A review of the literature. Australian Dental Journal. 2016;**61**:4-20

[3] Kindelan SA, Day PF, Kindelan JD, Spencer JR, Duggal MS. Dental trauma: An overview of its influence on the management of orthodontic treatment. Part 1. Journal of Orthodontics. 2008;**35**:68-78

[4] Schwartz-Arad D, Levin L, Ashkenazi M. Treatment options of untreatable traumatized anterior maxillary teeth for future use of dental implantation. Implant Dentistry. 2004;**13**:11-19

[5] Poi WR, CardosoLde C, de Castro JC, Cintra LT, Gulinelli JL, de Lazari JA. Multidisciplinary treatment approach for crown fracture and crown root fracture a case report. Dental Traumatology. 2007;**23**:51-55

[6] Owtad P, Shastry S, Papademetriou M, Park JH. Management guidelines for traumatically injured teeth during orthodontic treatment. The Journal of Clinical Pediatric Dentistry. 2015;**39**:292-296

[7] Bauss O, Röhling J, Meyer K, Kiliaridis S. Pulp vitality in teeth suffering trauma during orthodontic therapy. The Angle Orthodontist. 2009;**79**:166-171

[8] Al-Nazhan S, Andreasan JO, Al-Bawardi S, Al-Roug S. Evaluation of the effect of delayed management of traumatized permanent teeth. Journal of Endodontia. 1995;**21**:391-393

[9] Parkin SF. A recent analysis of traumatic injuries to children's teeth. Journal of Dentistry for Children. 1967;**34**:323-325

[10] Ravn JJ. Dental injuries in Copenhagen schoolchildren, school years 1967-1972. Community Dentistry and Oral Epidemiology. 1974;**2**:231-245

[11] Harrington MS, Eberhart AB, Knapp JF. Dentofacial trauma in children. Journal of Dentistry for Children. 1988;**55**:334-338

[12] Stock Well AJ. Incidence of dental trauma in the western Australian school dental service. Community Dentistry and Oral Epidemiology. 1988;**16**:294-298

[13] Perez R, Berkowitz R, McIlveen L, Forrester D. Dental trauma in children:A survey. Endodontics & Dental Traumatology. 1991;**7**:212-213

[14] Acton CHC, Nixon JW, Clark RC. Bicycle riding and oral/maxillofacial trauma in young children. The Medical Journal of Australia. 1996;**165**:249-251

[15] Galea H. An investigation of dental injuries treated in an acute care general hospital. Journal of the American Dental Association (1939). 1984;**109**:434-438

[16] Hamilton FA, Hill FJ, Holloway PJ. An investigation of dento-alveolar trauma and its treatment in an adolescent population. Part 1: The prevalence and incidence of injuries and the extent and adequacy of treatment received. British Dental Journal. 1997;**182**:91-95

[17] Hamilton FA, Hill FJ, Holloway PJ. An investigation of dento-alveolar trauma and its treatment in an adolescent population. Part 2: Dentists' knowledge of management methods and their perceptions of barriers to providing care. British Dental Journal. 1997;**182**:129-133

[18] Kostoupolou MN, Duggal MS. A study into dentist's knowledge of the treatment of traumatic injuries to young permanent incisors. International Journal of Paediatric Dentistry. 2005;**15**:10-19

[19] Kaste LM, Gift HC, Bhat M, Swango PA. Prevalence of incisor trauma in persons 6 to 50 years of age: United States, 1988-1991. Journal of Dental Research. 1996;**75**:696-705

[20] Andreasen J, Andreasen F, Andersson L. Traumatic Injuries to the Teeth. 4th ed. Copenhag: Blackwell publishing Company; 2007

[21] Bakland LK, Andreasen JO. Dental traumatology: Essential diagnosis and treatment planning. Endodontic Topics. 2004;**7**:14-34

[22] Shulman JD, Peterson J. The association between incisor trauma and occlusal characteristics in individuals 8-50 years of age. Dental Traumatology. 2004;**20**:67-74

[23] Newsome PR, Tran DC, Cooke MS. The role of the mouthguard in the prevention of sports-related dental injuries: A review. International Journal of Paediatric Dentistry. 2001;**11**:396-404

[24] Brin I, Ben-Bassat Y, Heling I, Engelberg A. The influence of orthodontic treatment on previously traumatized permanent incisors. European Journal of Orthodontics. 1991;**13**:372-377

[25] Turkistani J, Hanno A. Recent trends in the management of dentoalveolar traumatic injuries to primary and young permanent teeth. Dental Traumatology. 2011;**27**:46-54

[26] Bach N, Baylard JF, Voyer R. Orthodontic extrusion: Periodontal considerations and applications. Journal of the Canadian Dental Association. 2004;**70**(11):775-780

[27] Wickwire N, Mcneil M, Northon L, Duell R. The effects of tooth movement upon endodontically treated teeth. The Angle Orthodontist. 1974;**44**:235-242

[28] Hamilton R, Gutmann J. Endodontic-orthodontic relationships: A review of integrated treatment planning challenges. International Endodontic Journal. 1999;**32**:343-360

[29] Hunter M, Hunter B, Kingdon A, Addy M, Dummer P, Shaw W. Traumatic injury to predisposing factors related to traumatic injuries to permanent teeth. Swedish Dental Journal. 1993;**17**:183-190

[30] Turley P, Crawford L, Carrington K. Traumatically intruded teeth. The Angle Orthodontist. 1987;**57**:234-244

[31] Heithersay G. Combined endodontic-orthodontic treatment of transverse root fractures in the region of the alveolar crest. Oral Surgery, Oral Medicine, and Oral Pathology. 1973;**36**:404-415

[32] Malmgren O, Malmgren B, Frykholm A. Rapid orthodontic extrusion of crown root and cervical root fractured teeth. Endodontics & Dental Traumatology. 1991;**7**:49-54

[33] Flores MT, Andersson L, Andreasen JO, et al. Guidelines for the management of traumatic dental injuries. I. Fractures and luxations of permanent teeth. Dental Traumatology. 2007;**23**:66-71

[34] Fayle SA. Root fractures. In: Curzon MEJ, editor. Handbook of Dental Trauma. 1st ed. Boston: Wright; 1999. pp. 99-105

[35] Malmgren O, Malmgren B, Goldson L. Orthodontic management of the traumatised dentition. In: Andreasen JO, Andreasen FM, Andersson L, editors. Textbook and Color Atlas of Traumatic Injuries to the Teeth. 4th ed. Oxford: Blackwell Munksgaard; 2007. pp. 669-715

[36] Andreasen JO, Bakland LK, Matras RC, Andreasen FM. Traumatic intrusion of permanent teeth. Part 1: An epidemiological study of 216 intruded permanent teeth. Dental Traumatology. 2006;**22**:8-89

[37] Andreasen F, Andreasen J, Bayer T. Prognosis of root fractured permanent incisors- prediction of healing modalities. Endodontics & Dental Traumatology. 1989;**5**:11-22

[38] Malmgren O, Goldson L, Hill C, Orwin A, Petrini L, Lundberg M. Root resorption after orthodontic treatment of traumatized teeth. American Journal of Orthodontics and Dentofacial Orthopedics. 1982;**82**:487-491

[39] Seddon RP. Concomitant intrusive luxation and root fracture of a central incisor—Report of a case. Endodontics & Dental Traumatology. 1997;**13**:99-102

[40] Schöder U, Granath L. A new interceptive treatment of cases with missing maxillary lateral incisors. Swedish Dental Journal. 1981;**4**:155-158

[41] Slagsvold O, Bjercke B. Applicability of autotransplantation in cases of missing upper anterior teeth. American Journal of Orthodontics. 1978;**74**:410-421

[42] Czochrowska E, Skaare A, Stenvik A, Zachrisson B. Outcome of orthodontic space closure with a missing maxillary central incisor. American Journal of Orthodontics and Dentofacial Orthopedics. 2003;**123**:597-603

[43] Diaz J, Almeida M, Benavente A. Tooth transplantation after dental injury sequelae in children dent. Trauma. 2008;**24**:320-327

[44] Farahani A, Farahani B, Eslamipour F. An investigation into the association between facial profile and maxillary incisor trauma, a clinical non-radiographic study. Dental Traumatology. 2010;**26**:403-406

[45] Malmgren B, Malmgren O. Rate of infraposition of reimplanted ankylosed incisors related to age and growth in children and adolescents. Dental Traumatology. 2002;**18**:28-36

[46] Czochrowska EM, Skaare AB, Stenvik A, Zachrisson BU. Outcome of orthodontic space closure with a missing maxillary central incisor. American Journal of Orthodontics and Dentofacial Orthopedics. 2003;**123**:597-603

[47] Zachrisson BU, Stenvik A, Haanaes HR. Management of missing maxillary anterior teeth with emphasis on autotransplantation. American Journal of Orthodontics and Dentofacial Orthopedics. 2004;**126**:284-288

[48] Vilhjalmsson VH, Knudsen GC, Grung B, Bardsen A. Dental auto-transplantation to anterior maxillary sites. Dental Traumatology. 2011;**27**:23-29

[49] Andreasen J, Paulsen H, Bayer T. A long-term study of 370 autotransplanted premolars. Part IV, Root development subsequent to transplantation. European Journal of Orthodontics. 1990;**12**:38-50

[50] Roberts J, Olsen C, Messer H. Conservative management of an intruded immature maxillary permanent incisor with healing complication of pulp bone. Australian Endodontic Journal. 2001;**27**:29-32

[51] Shroff B. Canine impaction: Diagnosis, treatment planning, and clinical management. In: Nanda R, editor. Clinical Orthodontics. Philadelphia, PA: WB Saunders; 1997. pp. 99-108

[52] Graupner J. The effects of orthodontic force on replanted teeth: A radiographic survey. American Journal of Orthodontics. 1972;**62**:544-545

[53] Isaacson RJ, Strauss RA, Bridges-Poquis A, Peluso AR, Lindauer SJ. Moving an ankylosed central incisor using orthodontics, surgery and distraction osteogenesis. The Angle Orthodontist. 2001;**71**:411-418

[54] Kofod T, Wütz V, Melsen B. Treatment of an ankylosed central incisor by single tooth dento-osseous osteotomy and a simple distraction device. American Journal of Orthodontics and Dentofacial Orthopedics. 2005;**127**:72-80

[55] Chang HY, Chang YL, Chen HL. Treatment of a severely ankylosed central incisor and a missing lateral incisor by distraction osteogenesis and orthodontic treatment. American Journal of Orthodontics and Dentofacial Orthopedics. 2010;**138**:829-838

[56] Kokich VG, Crabill KE. Managing the patient with missing or malformed maxillary central incisors. American Journal of Orthodontics and Dentofacial Orthopedics. 2006;**129**(4 suppl):55-63

[57] Kawanami M, Andreasen J, Borum M, Schou S, Hjörting E, Kato H. Infraposition of ankylosed permanent maxillary incisors after replantation related to age and sex. Endodontics & Dental Traumatology. 1999;**15**:50-56

[58] Alcan T. A miniature tooth-borne distractor for the alignment of ankylosed teeth. The Angle Orthodontist. 2006;**76**:77-83

[59] Chae J, Paeng J. Orthodontic treatment of an ankylosed maxillary central incisor through single-tooth osteotomy by using interdental space regained from microimplant anchorage. American Journal of Orthodontics. 2012;**141**:39-51

[60] Malmgren B, Cvek M, Lundberg M, Frykholm A. Surgical treatment of ankylosed and infrapositioned reimplanted incisors in adolescents. Scandinavian Journal of Dental Research. 1984;**92**:391-399

[61] Andersson L. Dentoalveolar ankylosis and associated root resorption in replanted teeth. Experimental and clinical studies in monkeys and man. Swedish Dental Journal. Supplement. 1988;**56**:1-75

[62] Linge BO, Linge L. Apical root resorption in upper anterior teeth. European Journal of Orthodontics. 1983;**5**:173-183

[63] Levander E, Malmgren O, Eliasson S. Evaluation of root resorption in relation to two orthodontic treatment regimes. A clinical experimental study. European Journal of Orthodontics. 1994;**16**:223-228

[64] Levander E, Malmgren O. Long-term follow-up of maxillary incisors with severe apical root resorption. European Journal of Orthodontics. 2000;**22**(1):85-92

[65] Tsukiboshi M. Crown-Root Fracture. Treatment Planning for Traumatized Teeth. Quintessence Pub Co; 2000. p. 35, 45

[66] Reminghton D, Joondeph D, Arthun J, Riedel R, Chapko M. Long term evaluation of root resorption occurring during orthodontic treatment. American Journal of Orthodontics and Dentofacial Orthopedics. 1989;**98**:43-46

[67] Koroluk L, Tulloch J, Phillips C. Incisor trauma and early treatment for class II division 1 malocclusion.

American Journal of Orthodontics and Dentofacial Orthopedics. 2003;**123**:117-125

[68] Andersson L, Ermani Z, Högstrom J. Single tooth implant treatment in the anterior region of the maxilla for treatment of tooth loss after trauma :A retrospective clinical and interview study. Dental Traumatology. 2003;**19**:126-131

[69] Bowden D, Patel H. Autotransplantation of premolar teeth to replace missing maxillary central incisors. British Journal of Orthodontics. 1990;**17**:21-28

Section 7

Biochemistry

Chapter 7

Platelet-Rich Plasma in Trauma Patients

Mehmet Yaltirik, Meltem Koray, Hümeyra Kocaelli and Duygu Ofluoglu

Abstract

Platelet-rich plasma (PRP) was mixed with thrombin and excess calcium resulting in activated platelets trapped within the fibrin network; within the matrix, platelets secrete bioactive substances that diffuse into the surroundings tissues. PRP is prepared from the patient's own blood, a variety of manufacturing techniques in vastly different cell counts, and growth factor concentrations. The clinical use of PRP is treatment of soft tissue diseases and injuries, treatment of burns, hard-to-heal wounds, tissue engineering, and implantology in dentistry. An essential criterion for PRP is for it to be autologous, for the donor of the blood, and the recipient of the PRP to the same person. Most of the literatures suggest that PRP does not appreciably impact bone healing or induce bone formation. PRP might augment recruitment of osteoblast progenitors to injection sites or in sites expected to experience delayed healing. In this capacity, PRP might be utilized to initiate repair of an otherwise poorly healing bony lesion. PRP stimulates bone repair in fractures. Early through late healing process is compromised with fractures, including reduced cell proliferation, delayed chondrogenesis, and decreased biomechanical properties. In this chapter, the importance of the PRP in oral and maxillofacial surgery in trauma patients is studied

Keywords: platelet-rich plasma, trauma, oral surgery

1. Introduction

Today, regenerative therapy is the most preferred treatment because it is a method that meets the expectations of the patient close to the ideal. With the progress of technology, new materials about growth factors are entering our lives. Tissue engineering is currently working hard to develop regenerative materials. The health sector and tissue engineering benefit from each other in this respect.

First-generation platelet concentrate platelet-rich plasma (PRP) was used as a biomaterial to speed up the process of healing of the tissues. PRP contains high concentrations of platelets and growth factors in the low-volume plasma. These growth factors stimulate cell proliferation, matrix formation, and angiogenesis [1].

In 2001, platelet-rich fibrin (PRF), a second-generation platelet concentrate product, was developed in France, which was first developed for use in oral and maxillofacial surgery [2]. PRF preparation technique is based on the principle of collecting platelets and growth factors in the fibrin matrix by centrifuging venous blood from the patient. There are many forms of PRF materials such as P-PRF, L-PRF, A-PRF, I-PRF, and T-PRF used in oral and maxillofacial surgery.

2. Platelets

Platelets are cytoplasmic fragments of mature megakaryocytes in bone marrow. They are responsible for tissue regeneration by clotting, at the onset of wound healing, and by growth factors released from alpha granules. They are isolated from peripheral blood vessels [3].

Because of their short lifespan, the megakaryocytes should produce about $1.5–4 \times 10^{10}$ platelets per day to keep the platelet count in the normal blood count at $1.5–4.5 \times 10^5$ per microlitre (μL) of blood [4].

In 1960s, the interaction between platelets and endothelial cells supporting capillary endothelin integrity was revealed [5, 6]. Initial work by Folkman and colleagues used autologous PRP-augmented media to feed microvascular endothelial cells to enhance vascular integrity preservation in organs subjected to perfusion for transplantation. It has been determined that human platelet lysate (HPL) was prepared by repeated freezing/thawing cycles throughout the 1980s, and cell lines and primer fibroblasts were promoted by fresh blood or old platelet concentrates [7–9].

Platelets are quite active in terms of metabolism. Growth factors were released by platelet function with the phenomenon of "activation of macrophages by an increase in connective tissue healing, bone regeneration and repair, mitogenesis of fibroblasts, and angiogenesis of the wound area" by stimulating cell proliferation [10, 11].

After the resulting tissue damage, the platelets appear and the basal membrane of the collagen capillaries and the subendothelial microfibrils directly change shape. The alpha granules in the platelets engage the cell plasma membrane and release protein contents around with activation [11].

If the defects are small, platelet clotting is sufficient, and large wounds may require blood clots. The blood clot is activated from intrinsic and extrinsic pathways. "Intrinsic pathway" begins when there is a change in tissue damage or in blood. The "extrinsic pathway" begins with blood contact with factors other than blood, such as damaged tissue. Although they start differently in two ways, they converge on the next steps and share the reaction series. Coagulation in the presence of calcium and thrombin occurs by fibrinogen polymerization of fibrinogen monomers. The fibrin clot also provides a matrix environment for migration of fibroblasts and other tissue-forming cells, including endothelial cells, other than hemostasis [12].

3. Wound healing

Wound healing is a complex but a controlled mechanism regulated by growth factors and extracellular matrix.

Healing stages are:

1. hemostasis,

2. inflammation,

3. proliferation (granulation and contraction), and

4. remodeling (maturation) [13].

3.1 Hemostasis

Platelets behave like workers who close the damaged gas and water lines and seal damaged blood vessels. Blood vessels react to injury by vasoconstriction, but this spasm ends loosely. Thrombocytes secrete vasoconstrictor substances to facilitate this process, but this is not the main role. The primary role of platelets is to form clots. Adenosine diphosphate (ADP) leaks from damaged tissues. Platelets adhering to type 1 collagen, which is activated by ADP, thus become active. They are viscous glycoproteins that secrete and cause platelet aggregation [14]. At the same time, thrombocytes secrete factors that interact with and stimulate intracellular coagulation by intrinsic thrombin production, which initiates fibrinogen to fibrin. Platelets also secrete platelet-derived growth factors, known as one of the initiating factors for the healing process.

3.2 Inflammation

Inflammation is clinically associated with pain, swelling, temperature, and erythema, occurring between the first and fourth days after injury. Neutrophils perform their first defense against infection by phagocytosing existing debris and microorganisms. When the neutrophils digest bacteria and debris, they complete their task and die.

In wound repair, communication between soluble proteins and cells is ensured. These soluble proteins are growth factors and cytokines released by the cell. The role of the extracellular matrix in wound healing is activation of platelets, epithelial migration, and interaction with cells through receptors called integrins that lead to the movement of fibroblasts [15].

Macrophages secrete bacterial phagocytes and extracellular enzymes, to break down necrotic tissues and form the second line of defense. Secreted extracellular enzymes and matrix metalloproteinases (MMP) are calcium and zinc sources for the active site. MMP is responsible for necrotic tissue removal and repair of damaged tissue. MMP metalloproteinases are inactivated by tissue inhibitors (TIMPs) and uncontrolled activities are counterbalanced. Macrophages, fibroblast growth factor, epidermal growth factor, transforming growth factor-beta (TGF-β) and interleukin 1, etc. stimulate proliferation by secretion of cytokines and growth factors [16].

3.3 Proliferation

Proliferation begins after the injury of tissues and continues until the size of the wound and the systemic condition of the patient is up to 21 days in acute injuries. Characteristically, "angiogenesis," "collagen deposition," "granulation tissue" formation, "wound contraction," and "epithelialization" are seen at this stage.

Cells are introduced into the proliferation phase: macrophages, fibroblasts, pericytes, endothelial cells, and keratinocytes.

Fibroblasts are responsible for the secretion of collagen. In case of a damaged home, "plumber" cells are pericytes that renew outer layers of capillaries and endothelial cells that "glue." This process is called angiogenesis. Keratinocytes play the role of "roof plumber" and are responsible for epithelization.

3.4 Remodeling

Similarly, collagen tissue must be rearranged to provide greater tensile strength in wound repair. In addition, the density of cells and capillaries is reduced. The main cells involved in this process are fibroblasts. Remodeling can last up to 2 years after wounding [17].

4. Three therapeutic improvements through the wound healing mechanism: primary, secondary, and tertiary healing

4.1 Primary wound healing

Primary wound healing is called healing if the cleaved cleft is closed without any complications. Within 24 h, the minimal space existing between them is filled with fibrin and makes fibrinous adhesion.

4.2 Secondary wound healing

The healing form of granulation tissue in open wounds is called "secondary wound healing." Initially wounded with clots and exudates, the wound is filled by fibroblasts 4–5 days after injury. In this type of healing, the wound surface is covered with scar tissue after 30–40 days following injury.

4.3 Tertiary wound healing

In case of infection, in the over-devitalized tissues and in the presence of a foreign body, the improvement observed by closing the wound after a few days is called "delayed primary healing" (tertiary wound healing).

5. Platelet-rich plasma (PRP)

Platelet-rich plasma (PRP) was first developed in the early 1970s, but it was used rarely. PRP was mixed with thrombin and excess calcium resulting in activated platelets trapped within the fibrin network; within the matrix, platelets secrete bioactive substances that slowly diffuse into the surroundings tissues. PRP was introduced to the dental community by Whitman and colleagues, who hypothesized that the activation of platelets and the subsequent release of growth factors would enhance surgical healing [10]. PRP is now commonly applied to surgical sites and injuries to promote wound healing. PRP is rich in growth factors (PRGF), platelet-rich fibrin matrix (PRFM), and platelet-rich fibrin (PRF) [18].

The natural blood clot contains 95% of red blood cells, 5% of platelets, and 1% of white blood cells; thrombocyte-rich plasma obtained by centrifugation of blood tissue contains 4% of red blood cells, 95% of platelets, and 1% of white blood cells. Platelet concentrates in plasma are called "platelet-rich plasma." The goal of using platelet-rich plasma is to accelerate healing. High levels of platelets and growth factors also include all components of clotting factors. At least 5 ml of plasma is required for platelet-rich plasma to be clinically effective in order to have 10^6 μl of platelets. The platelet-rich plasma should be prepared in nonclotted form and should be used within 10 min from the start of coagulation [19, 20].

"Platelet-rich plasma" is administered by "injection" to the site of interest or by mixing with "grafts." "Platelet-rich plasma" has a long storage period, but should be used quickly when used. It takes up to 7 days in the region where the growth factors are applied [21].

1. Preparation of platelet-rich plasma

Nowadays, there are many preparation methods. These are as follows:

a. Preparation with standard blood bank procedures:
    - It can be prepared in Aferez units
    - It can be prepared from whole blood donors

2. It can be prepared with the aid of a test tube with 20–60 cc of blood.

3. It can be prepared using commercially available automatic preparation devices [22, 23].

4. PRP is subjected to a process known as differential centrifugation. It is prepared clinically by "PRP method" or "buffy coat method" [22, 23].

In the PRP method, an initial centrifuge (3000 rpm for 3 min) at low speed separates red blood cells (RBC), and then a second centrifuge (4000 rpm for 3 min) is applied at high speed to concentrate the platelets. In the initial centrifuge, the venous blood is centrifuged in tubes containing citrate dextrose. Acid citrate dextrose is an anticoagulant agent.

After the initial centrifugation, the whole blood is divided into three layers:

1. A top layer (platelet poor plasma) containing mostly "platelets" and "white blood cells (WBCs)" is of 40%.

2. An intermediate layer is rich in white blood cells known as the buffy coat and is of 5%.

3. A lower layer consisting mostly "red blood cells" is of 55% [23].

For the production of pure PRP (P-PRP), the top layer and the cover of the intermediate layer known as the buffy coat are transferred into an empty sterile tube. For the production of leucocyte-rich PRP (L-PRP), the top layer known as "PPP" is transferred to the entire layer of the "buffy coat" and a few "red blood cells." By the second centrifuge, the "red blood cells" and the PRP are separated. The PRP obtained after the second centrifugation is activated with thrombin and calcium chloride to prepare a PRP gel. PRP gel contains high amounts of platelets and natural fibrinogen. It takes approximately 30 min to prepare PRP with this technique. Prepared PRP should be used within 6 h.

6. Things to be aware of when preparing PRP

- In acid citrate dextrose (ACD-A), tubes should be obtained with whole blood by venipuncture.

- Blood should not be chilled at any time before platelet separation or platelet separation.

- Whole blood must first be centrifuged at "low speed."

- Supernatant containing platelets (floating on top of the precipitate) should be transferred into another sterile tube (no anticoagulant).

- Tube should be centrifuged at a higher speed (hard spin) to obtain platelet concentrate.

- At the end of centrifugation, bottom 1/3 of the tube consists of PRP and the top 2/3 consists of PPP. At the bottom of the tube platelet, pellets are observed.

- It is necessary to suspend platelet pellets in a minimum amount of plasma (2–4 ml) by removing the PPP and gently shaking the tube [24, 25].

There are also several factors that influence platelet concentration, such as the size of the platelets, the biological differences between individuals, and the hematocrit variability. It is more critical after the second centrifuge because the process of separating red blood cells intended for the first centrifugation may not be fully realized and erythrocytes may be present in the transferred volume. The remaining erythrocytes form a pellet at the base of the tube. Approximately, 20% of the platelets remain adsorbed on erythrocyte globules [26].

Another issue to be aware of is the impossibility of obtaining platelet-rich plasma from a non-anticoagulated blood. Platelets are responsible for the initiation of hemostasis and healing. Since platelets do not have platelets in the serum, it is not possible to obtain platelet-rich plasma from the serum, only anticoagulant platelets are possible.

Clinically, acid citrate dextrose or citrate phosphate dextrose is frequently used for anticoagulation. Citrate phosphate dextrose, acid citrate dextrose, has similar properties but has been suggested to be 10% less effective in protecting thrombocyte vitalites in studies. EDTA is not recommended because it will damage the platelet membrane.

Dual centrifugation technique is necessary to prepare platelet-rich plasma. Not enough platelets can be obtained with a single centrifugation and a mixture of both platelet-rich plasma and thrombocyte poor plasma cannot be separated completely [26].

7. Mechanism of action of platelet-rich plasma

Growth factors alone do not increase bone production. Platelets increase in the area applied with platelet-rich plasma. The increase in platelets also increases the growth factors numerically. PRP also contributes to bone regeneration by increasing the number of stem cells in a small number. Marx used a combination of bone graft and platelet-rich plasma in mandibular defects and attributed the contribution of platelet-rich plasma to bone regeneration to the function of growth factors in the environment [27].

Platelet-rich plasma is the basis for the activation of defense mechanisms by the activation of macrophages and the formation of a nonspecific immunoreaction with the leukocytes and interleukins involved.

The platelet-rich plasma has antimicrobial properties against microorganisms such as "*Escherichia coli,*" "*Staphylococcus aureus*," "*Candida albicans*," and "*Cryptococcus neoformans*" [28].

8. Duration of action and storage of platelet-rich plasma

The duration of action of PDGF and TGF-β in the platelet-rich plasma was investigated and a reduction in cell growth stimulating activity between 4 h and 3 days after venous blood ingestion was reported [29]. It is recommended to use PRP within the first 6 h after its preparation to keep the prepared biomaterials at a minimum level of contamination and to minimize disease transmission risks [30, 31]. It has been suggested that the degranulation of platelets and the release of growth factors are within the first 3–5 days; therefore, the effect of platelet-rich plasma is also 7–10 days [32]. Although the direct effects of platelets and growth factors are lost, bone regeneration is expected to continue, since the lifespan of active osteoblasts is approximately 3 months [33, 34].

9. Classification of platelet-derived blood concentrates

9.1 Pure platelet-rich plasma (P-PRP)

Using only the upper part of the yellowish layer to inhibit the presence of leukocytes, resulting biomaterial leads to a lower platelet count. Because it is possible to prepare clinically, it is a low-cost application [33, 35].

9.2 Leukocyte and platelet-rich plasma (L-PRP)

Blood in sterile tube containing no anticoagulants is subjected to initial centrifugation. All of the poor plasma and buffy coat layers from the cell and a portion of the bottom layer containing the red blood cells are transferred to a new tube. At a high speed, a second centrifugation is carried out and the poor plasma layer from the cell is withdrawn by pipetting. Coagulation is achieved by adding thrombin or calcium chloride as the activator. L-PRP, which takes time to prepare by hand, also has low density [35].

9.3 Pure platelet-rich fibrin (S-PRF)

The "P-PRP," "L-PRP," and "P-PRF" biomaterials all contain too much tombocytes from physiological values. It is reported in the literature that biomaterials with platelet content 2.5 times more than the number of platelets present are most effective [36].

9.4 Leukocyte and platelet-rich fibrin (Choukroun's PRF) (L-PRF)

L-PRF is a platelet concentrate containing all components of blood. There is no need for any anticoagulant agents in the preparation of L-PRF, so it can be regarded as a second-generation platelet concentrate. It is used in oral, maxillofacial, otorhinolaryngology, and plastic surgery. In the technique of preparing L-PRF, platelets and leukocytes are obtained with high efficiency. With the activation of L-thrombocytes, thrombocyte and leukocyte growth factors are embedded in the fibrin matrix [37–44]. In the biomaterial prepared, leukocytes act as an infection-preventive cells and immunomodulator [45, 46].

9.5 Advanced platelet-rich fibrin (A-PRF)

For L-PRF preparation, centrifugation for 12 min at a speed of 2700 rpm is required, but at a slower speed such as 1500 rpm for A-PRF preparation, longer time such as 14 min is required. Studies have shown that the number of viable cells, including platelets, is higher in A-PRF. Clinically, it will be beneficial for increasing amounts of growth factor and cytokine release. Reported that the levels of growth factors (TGF, PDGF-AB, VEGF) released from A-PRF are less than those of L-PRF when compared to that of L-PRF [47].

9.6 Injectable platelet-rich fibrin (I-PRF)

One of the latest developments in PRF technology is the production of injectable PRF (I-PRF). For preparation of I-PRF, blood samples are taken in plastic tube without anticoagulant and centrifuged at 2400–2700 rpm at about 700°C for 2–3 min [48].

9.7 Titanium platelet-rich fibrin (T-PRF)

During PRF preparation, different products are obtained using different materials for blood processing. Medical titanium tubes to produce PRF and 111333, named this material T-PRF [49]. In one study, it was observed that T-PRF samples had a fairly regular network than L-PRF samples [49]. In addition, the T-PRF fibrin network was observed to cover the wider area of the L-PRF fibrin network and the fibrin was thicker in the T-PRF specimens. T-PRF was obtained by centrifugation of 20 ml of blood at 2800 rpm for 12 min in medical titanium tubes in a human study. T-PRF membranes were found to have positive effects on palatal mucosal wound healing [49].

9.8 Concentrated growth factor (CGF)

The most important different CD34 stem cell content from the thrombocyte-rich plasma and fibrin of the concentrated growth factor is the content. CGF-CD34 is the name of the layer containing platelets, leukocytes, growth factors, and cytokines by separating the autologous blood into its components by centrifugation at four different rpm at the same time. Concentrated growth factor does not cause any infection or immunological reaction as it is prepared from the own blood of the person, and no chemicals are used during the process. CGF causes less inflammation, bleeding, and pain than other materials. Due to the stem cell content of CD34, regeneration capacity is higher than other biomaterials [50].

10. In vitro applications of thrombocyte-rich plasma

Although the clinical use of PRP and PRF is widespread in oral and maxillofacial surgery, the mechanism of cellular action has not yet been clearly elucidated. Although in vitro studies have been carried out on dental-derived cells, there is no comprehensive study describing the mechanism of action of stem cells. A limited number of in vitro studies do not provide a convenient and reliable basis for clinical practice.

Thrombin-activated plasma stimulate "adhesion," "migration," and "myofibroblastic differentiation" of human gingival fibroblasts [51]. In another study, PPP and 50% PRP resulted in the greatest increase in cellular proliferation and differentiation at various concentrations, the proliferation of osteoblast and periodontal connective tissue cells in platelet-rich plasma and platelet-poor plasma, and the effect on calcium formation [52].

Functions of the platelet-rich plasma are obtained from periodontal ligament tissue and pulp of human tooth root cells [53]. Colony formation and cellular proliferation of dental cells reduced platelet-rich plasma at concentrations of 0.5 and 1% [53].

Thrombocyte-rich fibrin regulates cell proliferation in a cell-type-specific manner, and that the thrombocyte-rich fibrin can promote cell proliferation [54].

In vitro studies of "platelet-rich plasma" have shown that the "PDGF-AB" and "TGF-β" factors are in high concentrations in platelet-rich plasma preparations and that the platelet—the proliferation [55, 56]. In another study of the same researchers, it was observed that the fibrinogen used with growth factors in platelet-rich plasma effectively increased wound healing in periodontal tissues.

11. Clinical studies on platelet-rich plasma

Contrary to in vitro studies, there is extensive literature in clinical trials. Thrombocyte-rich plasma in dentistry is used to increase tissue regeneration in periodontal disease, to accelerate healing of alveolar plugs after tooth extraction, and to accelerate osseointegration around dental implants [48, 56, 57].

First time, 88 mandibular bone defects were treated with autogenous bone graft, some with autogenous bone graft, and some with platelet-rich plasma. As a result of the study, it was observed that platelet-rich plasma significantly increased bone regeneration [27]. After tooth extraction, many complications can occur. There are studies showing that the graft site is covered with thrombocyte-rich plasma and local conditions such as "dry socket" and "abscess" formation are prevented, and conditions are improved. It has been reported that high aftertouch growth factor concentration increases tissue regeneration [58–62]. There are also studies in the literature, which show conflicting results with other studies suggesting that the platelet-rich plasma administered after tooth extraction does not have a significant effect. There are also observations that thrombocyte-rich plasma does not increase bone regeneration alone, as is the case with osseointegration at dental implant placement and studies that give positive platelet-rich plasma to accelerate new bone formation.

There are reports of positive results associated with thrombocyte-rich fibrin in sinus augmentation therapy prior to placement of the dental implant [62–66]. Co-use of deproteinized bovine bone (Bio-Oss) and thrombocyte-rich fibrin is only compared with Bio-Oss use; combined use of maxillary bone atrophy has been reported to give better results [67, 68].

Contradictory results have also been observed in the use of platelet-rich plasma in periodontal surgery. There are studies reporting increased tissue regeneration when applied with platelet-rich plasma graft materials [68, 69] while some studies suggest no improvement in healing process after thrombocyte-rich plasma implantation [70, 71]. The same conflicting results exist in the literature for thrombocyte-rich fibrin. Thrombocyte-rich fibrin in the third molar withdrawal of the mandible did not increase bone repair.

It has been demonstrated that the application of "thrombocyte-rich plasma" is effective in the "bison-linked osteonecrosis (BRONJ)" treatment of the jaw. The application of surgical debridement procedures in conjunction with autologous thrombocyte-rich plasma was reported that increased bone and soft tissue regeneration, increased neovascularization, and reduced tissue inflammation [71–76]. According to some investigators, thrombocyte-rich plasma regeneration capacity is a low biomaterial and may have a short-lived effect in the early phase of bone healing, flattening between the third and sixth months of treatment.

11.1 Use of platelet-rich plasma in surgical sockets

Thrombocyte-enriched plasma to the suction ports and stitch area of 170 patients after withdrawal of third molar teeth and alveolar osteitis was prevented with less pain and more intense bone formation [48].

In 20 patients with "periodontal defect" and "vertical root fracture" in two groups as thrombocyte-rich plasma and autogenous bone graft applied, only autogenous bone graft was applied. As a result, epithelialization of the group with autogenous bone grafting with thrombocyte-rich plasma and bone healing was faster [77].

11.2 Use of platelet-rich plasma in jaw reconstructions

"Autogenous bone graft" and "platelet-rich plasma" combination in "mandibular reconstruction" significantly improves bone healing [78]. Patients who underwent "partial mandibulectomy" combined "autogenous bone graft" and "thrombocyte-rich plasma" for reconstruction. After 6 months, they found that the biopsy bone they had received was sufficient and they applied the implant after 1 year [79].

11.3 Use of platelet-rich plasma in distraction osteogenesis

Implants in patients were done by injecting "mesenchymal stem cells" and "platelet-rich plasma" into the distraction range to obtain three-dimensional bones in the distraction osteogenesis of the mandible and to shorten the consolidation period. They reported that platelet-rich plasma was effective at the end of the study [80].

Injected mesenchymal stem cell and thrombocyte-rich plasma derived from bone marrow were used for "achondroplasia" and "congenital pseudoarthrosis. As a result of the study, they reported that short-term minimally invasive procedure is an advantage of increasing bone regeneration [81].

11.4 Use of platelet-rich plasma in individuals with alveolar cleft

Patients with alveolar congenital defects were using bone and tibia-derived grafts plus thrombocyte-rich plasma and reported that the corresponding region was rapidly restored according to the patient group, who had never used thrombocyte-rich plasma [82].

Autogenous bone grafts, in five of 12 patients with alveolar cleft, and the remaining seven were combined with autogenous bone and thrombocyte-enriched plasma in the remaining seven and closed the scales. They reported that regeneration in patients who were closed by a combination of autogenous bone and thrombocyte-rich plasma in a computed tomography scan was better than the other group [83].

11.5 Use of thrombocyte-rich plasma in oriented bone regeneration technique

Lecovic et al. reported that the combination of thrombocyte-rich plasma and bovine peroneal bone mineral was effective in the treatment of intrabony defects in patients with chronic periodontitis, although no directed tissue regeneration was performed [84].

11.6 Use of platelet-rich plasma after peripheral nerve injury

Peripheral nerve injuries may occur after surgical operations in the maxillofacial region and after trauma to the maxillofacial region. "Microsutures," "fibrin-cyanoacrylate adhesives," "grafting," and "laser" applications are preferred in the treatment of injured nerve tissue. However, the regenerative capacity of the nerve tissue is limited and heals very slowly. The use of platelet-rich plasma was considered to speed up this process of healing. An animal study was conducted using rats, although there is no human study on the subject. After the sciatic nerves of the rats were cut bilaterally, the nerve was connected with "cyanoacrylate" on one side and "platelet-rich plasma" on the other side. The number of nerve fibers formed on the treated side of the biopsied platelet-rich plasma after 12 weeks was higher than the other side [85].

11.7 Use of platelet-rich plasma in soft tissue injuries

Platelet-rich plasma is also effective in soft tissue injury as it is effective in hard tissue repair. Two groups were formed in the study in which 59 patients with acute traumatic soft tissue injury were treated. Thirty-two patients were treated with routine wound care while the remaining 27 patients were treated with routine thrombocyte-rich plasma as well as with routine wound healing. As a result, wound healing was faster in the platelet-rich plasma group [85].

12. Conclusion

Platelet-rich preparations are a safe (PRP) and is a preparation of plasma that contains an increased concentration of platelets compared to blood. PRP is autologous: for the recipient of the PRP to be the same person. PRP is used for both soft and hard tissue and also used in clinical dentistry, because it accelerates bone formation and induces healing.

Many studies support the use of autologous PRP in clinical practice, including for soft tissue injuries, chronic diabetic ulcers; injuries to muscles, tendons, or ligaments; bone fractures; molar extractions; urologic, dental, ophthalmic, and plastic surgery procedures; and periodontal, sinus lift, and oral/maxillofacial surgeries. Since growth factors play crucial roles in soft and hard tissue regeneration, the proposed mechanism for the enhanced healing outcomes by PRP is through the release of critical growth factors by activated platelets [86, 87].

Bone lesions and defects may arise out of many kinds of traumas. Due to the high prevalence of trauma, bone is the most transplanted tissue.

The use of autologous grafts is a gold standard to the biomaterial filling of bone defects. However, the limitation of tissue available, risks of infection, and necrosis re-motivated the proposition on synthetic biomaterials, which by turn are not biologically functional and adapted to remodeling bone tissue.

The use of biological factors, such as PRP and bone morphogenetic proteins (BMP), has shown good results in bone reconstructions, since they are directly associated with the tissues. Platelet growth factors such as platelet-derived growth factor (PDGF), transforming growth factor-b (TGF-b), fibroblast growth factor (FGF), vascular endothelial growth factor (VEGF)-A, and insulin-like growth factor (IGF-1) regulate bone regeneration, proliferation, and differentiation of osteoblasts, for the therapeutic use.

The use of PRP in the treatment of bone lesions has shown significant results from 1990s. PRP also used as an alternative to fibrin glue or platelet gel is frequently employed in maxillofacial defects. The therapeutic benefits and the reparative power of PRP consist of one action faster than conventional treatments maximized by autologous growth factors and are free from immune complications.

PRP action with the concentration of bone marrow had better consolidation and greater bone quantity by area in the PRP group. The superior result obtained can be explained by the immediate recruitment of all proteins necessary to start the healing cascade, while the concentration of bone marrow demanded longer time to recruit these elements. Thus, it can be assumed that the monitoring for a period of time up to 4 weeks, this group might have had similar results of consolidation. However, there were no new studies that could confirm this hypothesis.

Several studies reporting the association of PRP and artificial bone grafts showed improvement in the quality of healing. However, only PRP was used, and the short-term and/or long-term results, were positive but not significant. PRP could be beneficial and contribute to the morphological and functional improvement in chronic tendinopathy [86, 87].

In treatment of tendinopathy, PRP plays an important role. Physical therapy and a program of activities after injection of PRP, adopted in most studies, demonstrate better results in tendon lesions [88].

Platelet-rich plasma is a blood-derived product used for local healing. Interest in their activity over the last two decades has increased significantly in different disciplines. It is widely accepted that these materials stimulate soft and hard tissues to mimic the physiological healing process. The reason is that it contains high amounts of blood components such as fibrinogen, platelets, etc.

These biomaterials have been proposed for various uses in oral and maxillofacial surgery. Most studies in the literature: improvement of alveolar sockets after shrinkage, osseointegration of dental implants, sinus lifting procedures, improvement of periodontal bone defects, etc., examine the effects on the case. It has also been observed that platelet concentrations increase cell migration and neovascularization in vitro studies.

In addition to having many advantages of platelet-rich plasma, there are also disadvantages: increased risk of malign transformation as the PDGF release increases in chronic wounds, and the lack of factor V of the bovine thrombin used for anticoagulants and immunological reactions.

The activity of the platelet concentrates is expected with the high amounts of active growth factors and cytokines they contain. Nowadays, the preparation of these platelet concentrates is very different from each other. When platelet concentrates are compared, thrombocyte-rich fibrin is thought to have a higher regenerative potential than thrombocyte-rich plasma.

Platelet-rich plasma is a blood-derived product used for local healing. Interest in their activity over the last two decades has increased significantly in different disciplines. It is widely accepted that these materials stimulate soft and hard tissues to mimic the physiological healing process. The reason is that fibrinogen contains high amounts of blood components such as platelets.

Bone defects caused by infection, tumor, trauma, metabolic disease, or massive osteolysis due to prosthesis still remain a major clinical concern. Unfortunately, the self-repair capacity of the critically bone defected is extremely limited and this condition generally requires bone grafting. Osteoinductivity, osteoconductivity, and osteogenesis are optimal bone graft substitute. Allografts or xenografts have unique osteoconductive properties and rarely cause disease transmission. Because of these limitations, synthetic bone grafts are being used. Osteoinductive growth factors, autogenic bone marrow, and mesenchymal root cells promote osteogenesis while demineralized bone matrix (DBM) and platelet-rich plasma (PRP) induce formation of progenitor cells from surrounding tissues. However, each of these substitutes has its own significant limitations and none of them meets full expectations to serve as bone substitute in instance of bone defect.

Both PRP and DBM are osteoinductive substitutes that have shown satisfactory results for fracture healing. A number of growth and differentiation factors are liberated, including platelet-derived growth factor (PDGF), vascular endothelial growth factor (VEGF), transforming growth factor-1 (TGF-1), insulin-like growth factor-1 (IGF-1), hepatocyte growth factor, platelet factor-4, fibroblast growth factor (FGF), trombospondin-1, osteonectin, and fibronectin via activation of platelets. These factors play an important role in intracellular matrix formation, osteoid production, and the collagen synthesis involved in fracture healing. DBM is an organic collagen matrix that includes various types of bone morphogenetic proteins (BMP), which are responsible for its osteoinductive properties. PRP can be prepared easily with two-step centrifugation of autogenous blood, and DBM can be obtained commercially.

Through positive impacts of PRP and DBM based on these findings, the present study evaluated the impact of individual and combined applications of PRP and DBM on fracture healing of critical bone defects. Allogeneic PRP would have beneficial effect on treatment of segmental bone defects, comparable to DBM. Possibility of agonistic or additive osteoinductive effects of DBM and PRP combination was also investigated [89].

Despite the large number of clinical trial studies, there is little evidence of the cellular effect of blood derivatives. The lack of standard protocols leads to the lack of reliable clinical results. Frequent and unnecessary application of blood-derived products, especially in the maxillofacial region, results in both an increase in procedures and a significant increase in costs to clinicians and patients. The indications of the protocols for the application and preparation of blood derivatives should be made absolutely widespread and systematic in order to clarify the benefits for patients of blood derivatives. This can be achieved through a collaborative work between clinical and in vitro researchers. Further research on thrombocyte-rich plasma and thrombocyte-rich fibrin activity on dental cell biology, more clinical application of platelet concentrates, and greater use in the oral and maxillofacial region may provide a stable basis for more predictable outcomes.

Conflict of interest

We declare that there is no conflict of interest with any financial organization regarding the material discussed in the chapter.

Author details

Mehmet Yaltirik*, Meltem Koray, Hümeyra Kocaelli and Duygu Ofluoglu

Department of Oral and Maxillofacial Surgery, Faculty of Dentistry, Istanbul University, Istanbul, Turkey

*Address all correspondence to: mehmet.yaltirik@istanbul.edu.tr

References

[1] Graziani F, Ivanovski S, Cei S, Ducci F, Tonetti M, Gabriele M. The in vitro effect of different PRP concentrations on osteoblasts and fibroblasts. Clinical Oral Implants Research. 2006;**17**(2):212-219

[2] McCauley LK, Somerman MJ. Biologic modifiers in periodontal regeneration. Dental Clinics of North America. 1998;**42**(part I):361-386

[3] Marx RE, Carlson ER, Eichstaedt RM, et al. Platelet-rich plasma: Growth factor enhancement for bone grafts. Oral Surgery, Oral Medicine, Oral Pathology, Oral Radiology, and Endodontics. 1998;**85**:638-646

[4] Dohan Ehrenfest DM, Rasmusson L, Albrektsson T. Classification of platelet concentrates: From pure plateletrich plasma (P-PRP) to leucocyte- and platelet-rich fibrin (LPRF). Trends in Biotechnology. 2009;**27**:158-167

[5] Mishra A, Woodall J, Vieria A. Treatment of tendon and muscle using platelet rich plasma. Clinics in Sports Medicine. 2009;**28**(1):113-125

[6] Raghoebar GM, Schortinghuis J, Liem RSB, Ruben JL, Van Der Wal JE, Vissink A. Does platelet-rich plasma promote remodeling of autologous bone grafts used for augmentation of the maxillary sinus floor? Clinical Oral Implants Research. 2005;**16**:349-356

[7] Clark R. Fibrin glue for wound repair: Facts and fancy. Thrombosis and Haemostasis. 2003;**90**:1003-1006

[8] Kim SG, Chung C, Kim K, Park J. Use of particulate dentinplaster of Paris combination with/without platelet-rich plasma in the treatment of bone defects a round implants. The International Journal of Oral & Maxillofacial Implants. 2002;**17**:86-94

[9] Parker MH, Kuru L, Giouzeli M, Olsen I. Expression of growth-factor receptors in normal and regenerating human periodontal cells. Archives of Oral Biology. 2001;**46**:275-284

[10] Zimmermann R, Jakubietz R, Jakubietz M, Strasser E, Schlegel A, Wiltfang J, et al. Different preparation methods to obtain platelet components as a source of growth factors for local aplication. Transfusion. 2001;**41**:1217-1224

[11] Dohan DM, Del Corso M, Diss A, Mouhyi J, Charrier JB. Three-dimensional architecture and cell composition of a Choukroun's platelet-rich fibrin clot and membrane. Journal of Periodontology. 2010;**81**(4):546-555

[12] Nachman RL, Rafii S. Platelets, petechiae, and preservation of the vascular wall. The New England Journal of Medicine. 2008;**359**:1261-1270

[13] Burnouf T, Lee CY, Luo CW, et al. Human blood derived fibrin releasates: Composition and use for the culture of cell lines and human primary cells. Biologicals. 2012;**40**:21-30

[14] Landesberg R, Roy M, Glickman RS. Quantification of growth factor levels using a simplified method of platelet-rich plasma gel preparation. Journal of Oral and Maxillofacial Surgery. 2000;**58**:297-301

[15] Cáceres M, Hidalgo R, Sanz A, Martínez J, Riera P, Smith PC. Effect of platelet-rich plasma on cell adhesion, cell migration, and myofibroblastic differentiation in human gingival fibroblasts. Journal of Periodontology. 2008;**79**(4):714-720

[16] Fujita T, Shiba H, Van Dyke TE, Kurihara H. Differential effects of growth factors and cytokines on the

synthesis of SPARC, DNA, fibronectin and alkaline phosphatase activity in human periodontal ligament cells. Cell Biology International. 2004;**28**:281-286

[17] Lundquist R, Dziegiel MH, Agren MS. Bioactivity and stability of endogenous fibrogenic factors in platelet-rich fibrin. Wound Repair and Regeneration. 2008;**16**:356-363

[18] Ferreira FC, Gomez MCC, Filho JS, Granjeiro JM, Simoes CMO, Magini RS. Platelet-rich plasma influence on human osteoblasts growth. Clinical Oral Implants Research. 2005;**16**:456-460

[19] Chang KM, Lehrhaupt N, Lin LM, Feng J, Wu-Wang CY, Wang SL. Epidermal growth factor in gingival crevicular fluid and its binding capacity in inflamed and non-inflamed human gingiva. Archives of Oral Biology. 1996;**41**(7):719-724

[20] Anitua E, Andía I, Sanchez M, Azofra J, del Mar Zalduendo M, de la Fuente M, Nurden P, Nurden AT. Autologous preparations rich in growth factors promote proliferation and induce VEGF and HGF production by human tendon cells in culture. Journal of Orthopaedic Research. 2005;**23**(2):281-286

[21] Matsuda N, Lin WL, Kumar NM, Cho MI, Genco RJ. Mitogenic, chemotactic and synthetic responses of rat periodontal ligament fibroblastic cells to polypeptide growth factors in vitro. Journal of Periodontology. 1992;**63**:515-525

[22] Creeper F, Lichanska AM, Marshall RI, et al. The effect of platelet-rich plasma on osteoblast and periodontal ligament cell migration, proliferation and differentiation. Journal of Periodontal Research. 2009;**44**:258-265

[23] Ogundipe OK, Ugboko VI, Owotade FJ. Can autologous platelet rich plasma gel enhance healing after surgical extraction of mandibular third molars? Journal of Oral and Maxillofacial Surgery. 2011;**69**:2305-2310

[24] Anitua E, Aguirre JJ, Algorta J, Ayerdi E, Cabezas AI, Orive G, et al. Effectiveness of autologous preparation rich in growth factors for the treatment of chronic cutaneous ulcers. Journal of Biomedical Materials Research. Part B, Applied Biomaterials. 2008;**84**:415-421

[25] Dugrillon A, Eichler H, Kern S, Klüter H. Autologous concentrated platelet-rich plasma (cPRP) for local application in bone regeneration. International Journal of Oral and Maxillofacial Surgery. 2002;**31**:615-619

[26] Arenaz-Bua J, Luaces-Rey R, Sironvalle-Soliva S, et al. A comparative study of platelet-rich plasma, hydroxyapatite, demineralized bone matrix and autologous bone to promote bone regeneration after mandibular impacted third molar extraction. Medicina Oral, Patología Oral y Cirugía Bucal. 2010;**15**:483-489

[27] Diss A, Dohan DM, Mouhyi J, et al. Osteotome sinus floor elevation using Choukroun's platelet-rich fibrin as grafting material: A 1-year prospective pilot study with microthreaded implants. Oral Surgery, Oral Medicine, Oral Pathology, Oral Radiology, and Endodontics. 2008;**105**:572-579

[28] IntiniI G. The use of platelet rich plasma in bone reconstruction threapy. Biomaterials. 2009;**30**:4956-4966

[29] Choukroun J, Diss A, Simonpieri A, et al. Platelet-rich fibrin (PRF): A second-generation platelet concentrate. Part V: Histologic evaluations of PRF effects on bone allograft maturation in sinus lift. Oral Surgery, Oral Medicine, Oral Pathology, Oral Radiology, and Endodontics. 2006;**101**:299-303

[30] Braccini F, Dohan DM. The relevance of Choukroun's plateler rich

fibrin (PRF) during facial esthetic lipostructure (Coleman's technique): Preliminary results. Revue de Laryngologie Otologie Rhinologie. 2007;**128**(4):255-260

[31] Bausset O, Giraudo L, Veran J, Magalon J, Coudreuse JM, Magalon G, et al. Formulation and storage of platelet-rich plasma homemade product. BioResearch Open Access. 2012;**1**:115-123

[32] Hanson SR, Slichter SJ. Platelet kinetics in patients with bone marrow hypoplasia: Evidence for a fixed platelet requirement. Blood. 1985;**66**:1105-1109

[33] Dohan DM, Choukroun J, Diss A, et al. Platelet-rich fibrin (PRF): A second-generation platelet concentrate, part I: Technological concept and evolution. Oral Surgery, Oral Medicine, Oral Pathology, Oral Radiology, and Endodontics. 2006;**101**:37-44

[34] Schüppbach P, Gaberthüel T, Lutz F, Guggenheim B. Periodontal repair or regeneration: Structures of different types of new attachment. Journal of Periodontal Research. 1993;**28**:281-293

[35] Dohan S, Dohan A, Choukroun J, et al. De l'usage des concentrés plaquettaires autologues en application topique. L'Odontologie. 2005;**1**:141-180

[36] Kuru L, Griffiths GS, Petrie A, Olsen I. Changes in transforming growth factor-beta1 in gingival crevicular fluid following periodontal surgery. Journal of Clinical Periodontology. 2004;**31**:527-533

[37] Terranova VP, Odziemiec C, Tweden KS, Spadone DP. Repopulation of dentin surfaces by periodontal ligament cells and endothelial cells. Effect of basic fibroblast growth factor. Journal of Periodontology. 1989;**60**:293-301

[38] Hauschka PV, Mavrakos AE, Isafrati MD, Doleman SE, Klagsburn M. Growth factors in bone matrix. Isolation of multiple types by affinity chromatography on heparin-sepharose. The Journal of Biological Chemistry. 1986;**261**:12665-12674

[39] Callens A. Growth factors in periodontal regeneration. In: Lang NP, Karring T, Lindhe J, editors. Chemicals in Periodontics. Chicago IL: Quintessence; 1997. pp. 284-302

[40] Carlson NE, Roach RB. Platelet-rich plasma: Clinical applications in dentistry. Journal of the American Dental Association (Chicago, IL). 2002;**133**:1383-1386

[41] Oates TW, Rouse CA, Cochran DL. Mitogenic effects of growth factors on human periodontal ligament cells in vivo. Journal of Periodontology. 1993;**64**:142-148

[42] Slichter SJ. Relationship between platelet count and bleeding risk in thrombocytopenic patients. Transfusion Medicine Reviews. 2004;**18**:153-167

[43] Tweden KS, Spadone DP, Terranova VP. Neovascularization of surface demineralized dentin. Journal of Periodontology. 1989;**60**:460-466

[44] Bayan LA, Bhargava G, Nishimura F, Orman R, Price R, Terranova VP. Mitogenic and chemotactic responses of human periodontal ligament cells to the different isoforms of platelet derived growth factor. Journal of Dental Research. 1994;**73**:1593-1600

[45] Tajima Y, Yokose S, Koshimata M, Hiramatsu M, Minami N, Utsumi N. Epidermal growth factor expression in junctional epithelium of rat gingiva. Journal of Periodontal Research. 1992;**27**:299-300

[46] Slapnicka J, Fassmann A, Strasak L, Augustin P, Vanek J. Effects of activated and nonactivated

platelet-rich plasma on proliferation of human osteoblasts in vitro. Journal of Oral and Maxillofacial Surgery. 2008;**66**(2):297-301

[47] Mintz PD, Mayers L, Avery N, et al. Fibrin sealant: Clinical use and the development of the University of Virginia tissue adhesive center. Annals of Clinical and Laboratory Science. 2001;**31**:108-118

[48] Weibrich G, Hansen T, Kleis W, Buch R, Hitzler WE. Effect of platelet concentration in platelet-rich plasma on peri-implant bone regeneration. Bone. 2004;**34**(4):665-671

[49] Berberoğlu A. Periodontal Dokuların İyileşmesinde Büyüme Faktörlerinin Rolü. Hacettepe Dişhekimliği Fakültesi Dergisi. 2007;**3**:114-121

[50] Kerstein MD. The scientific basis of healing. Advances in Wound Care. 1997;**10**:30-36

[51] Dereka XE, Markopoulou CE, Vrotsos IA. Role of growth factors on periodontal repair. Growth Factors. 2006;**24**:260-267

[52] Zechner W, Tangl S, Tepper G, Fürst G, Bernhart T, Haas R, Mailath G, Watzek G. Influence of platelet-rich plasma on osseous healing of dental implants: A histologic and histomorphometric study in minipigs. The International Journal of Oral & Maxillofacial Implants. 2003;**18**(1):15-22

[53] King GL, Buchwald S. Characterization and partial purification of an endothelial cell growth factor from human platelets. The Journal of Clinical Investigation. 1984;**73**:392-396

[54] Burwell RC. Studies in the transplantation of bone. VII. The fresh composite homograft autograft of cancellous bone. An analysis of factors leading to osteogenesis in marrow transplantas and in marrowcontaining bone grafts. Journal of Bone and Joint Surgery. British Volume (London). 1964;**46-B**:110-140

[55] Boyapati L, Wang LH. The role of platelet-rich plasma in sinus augmentation: A critical review. Implant Dentistry. 2006;**15**:160-170

[56] Sweeny J, Grossman BJ. Blood collection, storage and component preparation methods. In: Brecher M, editor. Technical Manual. 14th ed. Bethesda MD: American Association of Blood Banks (AABB); 2002. pp. 955-958

[57] Plachokova AS, Nikolidakis D, Mulder J, Jansen JA, Creugers NH. Effect of platelet rich plasma on bone regeneration in dentistry: A systemic review. Clinical Oral Implants Research. 2008;**19**:539-545

[58] Position Paper. The potential role of growth and differentiation factors in periodontal regeneration. Journal of Periodontology. 1996;**67**:545-553

[59] Anitua E. Plasma rich in growth factors: Preliminary results of use in the preparation of future sites for implants. The International Journal of Oral & Maxillofacial Implants. 1999;**14**(4):529-535

[60] Sahni A, Odrljin T, Francis CW. Binding of basic fibroblast growth factor to fibrinogen and fibrin. The Journal of Biological Chemistry. 1998;**273**(13):7554-7559

[61] Cochran DL, Wozney JM. Biological mediators for periodontal regeneration. Periodontology 2000. 1999;**19**:40-58

[62] Gresele P, Page PC, Fuster V, Vermylen J, editors. Platelets in Thrombotic and Non-Thrombotic Disorders Pathophysiology,

Pharmacology and Therapeutics. Cambridge University Press; 2002. p. 25

[63] Field FK, Kerstein MD. Overview of wound healing in a moist environment. American Journal of Surgery. 1994;**167**(Suppl 1A):2S-6S

[64] Lozada JL, Caplanis N, Proussaefs P, Willardsen J, Kammeyer G. Platelet-rich plasma application in sinus graft surgery: Part I—Background and processing techniques. The Journal of Oral Implantology. 2001;**27**:38-42

[65] Krasna M, Domanović D, Tomsic A, Svajger U, Jeras M. Platelet gel stimulates proliferation of human dermal fibroblasts in vitro. Acta Dermatovenerologica Alpina, Panonica, et Adriatica. 2007;**16**(3):105-110

[66] Chang IC, Tsai CH, Chang YC. Platelet-rich fibrin modulates the expression of extracellular signal-regulated protein kinase and osteoprotegerin in human osteoblasts. Journal of Biomedical Materials Research. Part A. 2010; **95**(1):327-332

[67] Takayama S, Murakami S, Shimabukuro Y, Kitamura M, Okada H. Periodontal regeneration by FGF2 (bFGF) in primate models. Journal of Dental Research. 2001;**80**:2075-2079

[68] Grageda E. Platelet-rich plasma and bone graft materials: A review and a standardized research protocol. Implant Dentistry. 2004;**13**:301-309

[69] Choukroun JI, Braccini F, Diss A, et al. Influence of platelet rich fibrin (PRF) on proliferation of human preadipocytes and tympanic keratinocytes: A new opportunity in facial lipostructure (Coleman's technique) and tympanoplasty? Revue de Laryngologie Otologie Rhinologie. 2007;**128**:27-32

[70] Cenni E, Ciapetti G, Pagani S, Perut F, Giunti A, Baldini N. Effects of activated platelet concentrates on human primary cultures of fibroblasts and osteoblasts. Journal of Periodontology. 2005;**76**(3):323-328

[71] Matras H, Dinges H, Lassmann H, et al. Zur Nahtlosen interfaszikularen nerven transplantation im tierexperiment. Wiener Medizinische Wochenschrift. 1972;**112**:517-523

[72] Cafesse R, Quinones CR. Polypeptide growth factors and attachment proteins in periodontal wound healing and regeneration. Periodontology 2000. 1993;**1**:69-79

[73] Canalis E, Pash J, Gabbitas B, Rydziel S, Vargehese S. Growth factors regulate the synthesis of insulin-like growth factor-I in bone cell cultures. Endocrinology. 1993;**133**:33-38

[74] Han J, Meng HX, Tang JM, Li SL, Tang Y, Chen ZB. The effect of different platelet-rich plasma concentrations on proliferation and differentiation of human periodontal ligament cells in vitro. Cell Proliferation. 2007;**40**:241-252

[75] Jo CH, Roh YH, Kim JE, Shin S, Yoon KS. Optimizing platelet-rich plasma gel formation by varying time and gravitational forces during centrifugation. The Journal of Oral Implantology. 2013;**39**:525-532

[76] Parkar MH, Kuru L, Fgiouzeli M, Olsen I. Expression of growth factor receptors in normal and regenerative human periodontal cells. Archives of Oral Biology. 2001;**46**:679-688

[77] Epply BL, Pietrzak WS, Blanton M. Platelet-rich plasma. A review of biology and applications in plastic

surgery. Plastic and Reconstructive Surgery. 2006;**118**:147e-159e

[78] Waters JH, Roberts KC. Database review of possible factors influencing point-of-care platelet gel manufacture. The Journal of Extra-corporeal Technology. 2004;**36**:250-254

[79] Clausen C, Hermund NU, Donatsky O, Nielsen H, Osther K. Homologous activated platelets stimulate differentiation and proliferation of primary human bone cells. Cells, Tissues, Organs. 2006;**184**(2):68-75

[80] De Ranieri A, Virdi AS, Kurado S, Shott S, Leven RM, Hallab NJ, et al. Local application of rhTGFbeta2 enhances peri-implant bone volume and bone-implant contact in a rat model. Bone. 2005;**37**:55-62

[81] Welsh WJ. Autologous platelet gel: Clinical function and usage in plastic surgery. Cosmetic Dermatology. 2000;**11**:13-19

[82] Nordlund L, Hormia M, Saxen L, Thesleff I. Immunohistochemical localization of epidermal growth factor receptors in human gingival epithelia. Journal of Periodontal Research. 1991;**26**:333-338

[83] Braccini F, Dohan DM. The relevance of Choukroun's platelet rich fibrin (PRF) during facial aesthetic lipostructure (Coleman's technique): Preliminary results. Revue de Laryngologie Otologie Rhinologie. 2007;**128**:255-260

[84] Lekovic V, Milinkovic I, Aleksic Z, Jankovic S, Stankovic P, Kenney EB, Camargo PM. Platelet-rich fibrin and bovine porous bone mineral vs. platelet-rich fibrin in the treatment of intrabony periodontal defects. Journal of Periodontal Research. 2012;**47**:409-417

[85] Hussain N, Johal H, Bhandari M. An evidence-based evaluation on the use of platelet rich plasma in orthopedics—A review of the literature. SICOT J. 2017;**3**:57

[86] Davis VL, Abukabda AB, Radio NM, Witt-Enderby PA, Clafshenkel WP, Cairone JV, Rutkowski JL. Platelet-rich preparations to improve healing. Part II: Platelet activation and enrichment, leukocyte inclusion, and other selection criteria. Journal of Oral Implantology. 2014;(4):511-521

[87] Davis VL, Abukabda AB, Radio NM, Witt-Enderby PA, Clafshenkel WP, Cairone JV, Rutkowski JL. Platelet-rich preparations to improve healing. Part I: Workable options for every size practice. Journal of Oral Implantology. 2014;**4**:500-510

[88] Marques LF, Stessuk T, Camargo IC, Sabeh N Jr, dos Santos L, Ribeiro-Paes JT. Platelet-rich plasma (PRP): Methodological aspects and clinical applications. Platelets. 2015;**26**(2):101-113

[89] Egemen T, Mustafa KA, Ahmet B, Murat S, Selçuk K, Mahmut ND. A comparison of the effects of platelet-rich plasma and demineralized bone matrix on critical bone defects: An experimental study on rats. Ulusal Travma ve Acil Cerrahi Dergisi. 2017;**23**(2):91-99

Section 8

Soft Tissue Trauma

Chapter 8

Oral Mucosal Trauma and Injuries

Meltem Koray and Tosun Tosun

Abstract

Trauma-related oral lesions are common in clinical practice of dentistry and they can impair patients' normal oral function and cause pain in patients' eating, chewing, and talking. An injury to the oral mucosa can result from physical, chemical, or thermal trauma. Such injuries can result from accidental tooth bite, hard food, sharp edges of the teeth, hot food, or excessive tooth brushing. Some injuries can also be caused by iatrogenic damage during dental treatment or other procedures related to oral cavity. In this chapter, oral mucosal trauma and injuries will be examined in four subclasses: physical and mechanical traumas of oral mucosa; chemical injuries of the oral mucosa; radiation injuries; and electrical, thermal burns.

Keywords: trauma, soft tissue injuries, mucosa, traumatic injuries

1. Introduction

Trauma-related oral lesions are common in clinical practice of dentistry. Such lesions can impair patients' normal oral function and can cause pain in patients' eating, chewing, and talking. After receiving a diagnosis with anamnesis, treatment can be provided if the causative factor is removed. An injury to the oral mucosa can result from physical, chemical, or thermal trauma. Such injuries can result from accidental tooth bite, hard food, sharp edges of the teeth, hot food, or excessive tooth brushing. Some injuries can also be caused by iatrogenic damage during dental treatment or other procedures related to oral cavity [2]. This section focuses on common causes, diagnoses, and treatment of traumatic injuries. In the following, a proposed classification of oral mucosal trauma and injuries is described:

Classification of oral mucosal trauma and injuries:

A. Physical and mechanical traumas of oral mucosa

1. Linea alba
2. Chronic biting
3. Epulis fissuratum
4. Inflammatory papillary hyperplasia
5. Denture stomatitis
6. Traumatic ulcer
7. Recurrent aphthous stomatitis

8. Nicotine stomatitis
9. Lip-licking dermatitis
10. Traumatic fibroma
11. Trauma associated with sexual practice

B. Chemical injuries of the oral mucosa

1. Chemical burn
2. Post-anesthetic ulceration of palate
3. Contact allergic stomatitis

C. Radiation injuries

1. Oral mucositis
2. Actinic chellitis

D. Electrical and thermal burn

1. Electrical burn
2. Thermal burn

2. Physical and mechanical traumas of oral mucosa

2.1 Linea alba (white line)

Localization: Buccal mucosa, at the level of the occlusal line of the teeth. It is a horizontal streak on the buccal mucosa at the level of the occlusal plane extending from the commissure to the posterior teeth.

Clinical features: Lesions are mostly asymptomatic. The common visual symptom of linea alba is the presence of whitish, linear, filament-like plicae formations, horizontally parallel to the occlusal level of bicuspids and molar teeth in both left and right sides of buccal mucosa (**Figure 1**). Palpation should give a tactile sensation of normal mucosa texture. It is more prominent in individuals with reduced overjet of the posterior teeth. It is often scalloped and restricted to dentulous areas. The diagnosis is based on clinical grounds alone [11].

Etiology: Lesions mainly arise from occlusal traumas of posterior teeth generated due to the parafunctional cheek sucking of patient. The sucking habit is also associated with friction between buccal tubercules and irritates the buccal mucosa by pressure. Prevalence of such lesions is about 6.2–13% in the population [4, 5, 9].

Treatment: No treatment is required; the white streak may disappear spontaneously in some people. But very sharp-edged teeth can be corrected.

2.2 Chronic biting (*Morsicatio buccarum*)

Localization: The lesions made by chronic bite trauma (nibbling) on the buccal mucosa generally cause keratinized shreds, tissue tags, or erosive and desquamative surfaces [20]. These lesions according to their localizations are called as "morsicatio buccarum" if they are localized on the buccal mucosa, "morsicatio labiorum" if they

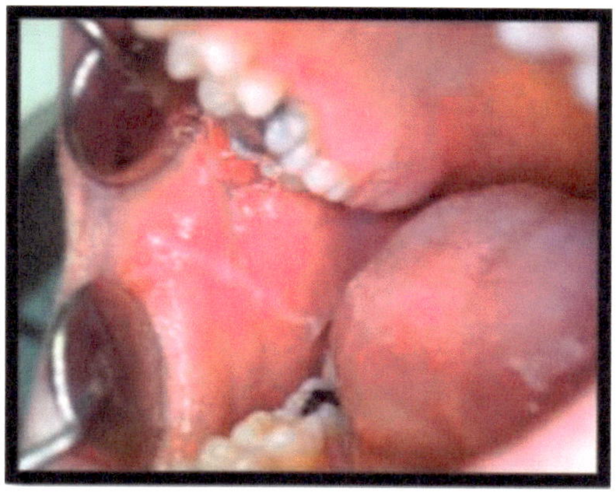

Figure 1.
Linea alba seen on the buccal mucosa.

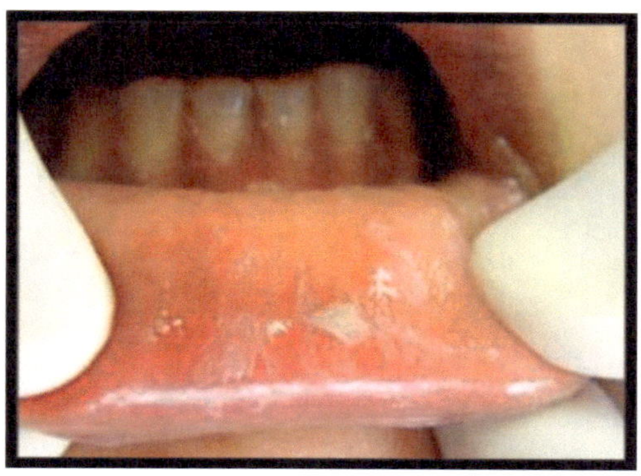

Figure 2.
Diffuse irregular white area of lower lip due to chronic biting.

appear on the labial mucosa, and "morsicatio linguarum" if they occur on the lateral borders of the tongue [21]. The lesions are seen on the buccal mucosa, bilateral chewing line, labial mucosa, and lateral edges of the tongue.

Clinical features: Lesions are apparent as shallow whitish wrinkles which are diffuse and present irregularly on the buccal, labial mucosa, and tongue. Epithelial desquamation occurs on the surface (**Figures 2** and **3**). In some cases, erosions and petechiae may be seen. The lesions could be diagnosed by clinical inspection [11].

Etiology: It is often related to chronic biting of the oral mucosa seen in psychologically tense patients. Parafunctional bite of the buccal mucosa, lips, and tongue until wear of superficial epithelium and wound formation is consciously made by those patients. The incidence of morsicatio buccarum was reported to be 2.5% in Caucasian populations [16].

Treatment: Treatment is usually unnecessary. It is recommended to stop the habit. Psychological treatment can be suggested for stopping a bad habit. Acrylic splint can be made on the occlusal surface of the teeth. It is accepted as a precancerous lesion.

2.3 Epulis fissuratum

Localization: The lesion presents as multiple or single inflamed and elongated papillary folds, usually in the mucolabial or mucobuccal grooves around poorly fitting partial or complete denture.

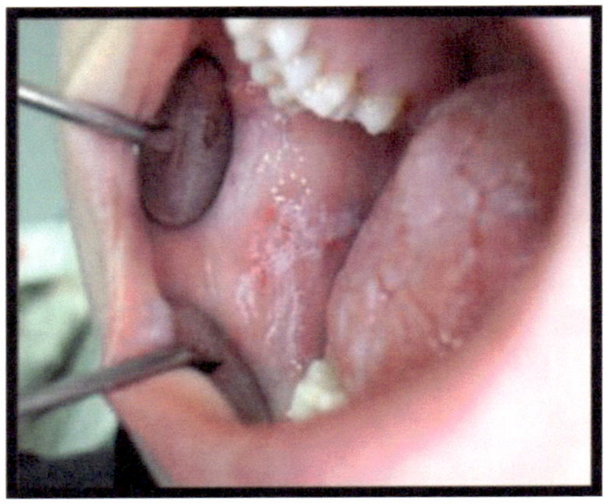

Figure 3.
Chronic biting of the buccal mucosa with diffuse irregular lesions.

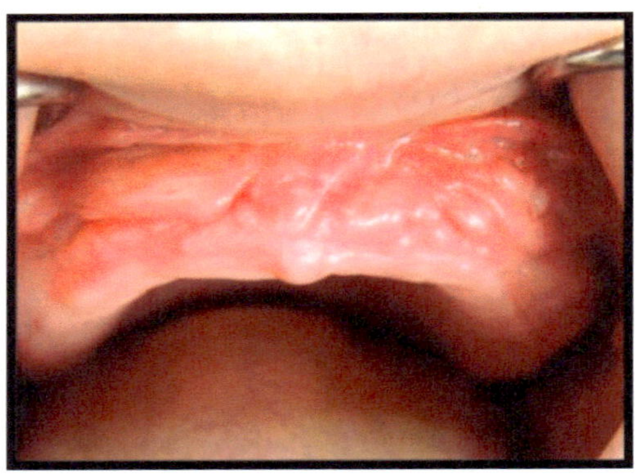

Figure 4.
Epulis fissuratum.

Clinical features: Epulis fissuratum, reactive fibrous hyperplasia, or denture-induced fibrous hyperplasia is a relatively common hyperplasia of the fibrous connective tissue. Clinically, it presents as a raised sessile lesion in the form of folds with a smooth surface with normal or erythematous overlying mucosa. Because of chronic irritation, it may get traumatized and present with an ulcerated surface. It is considered as an overgrowth of intraoral tissues resulting from chronic irritation. This mucogingival hyperplasia is a reactive condition of oral mucosa to excessive mechanical pressure on mucosa (**Figure 4**).

Etiology: Trauma and irritation are the two main etiological factors responsible for occurrence of epulis. It is attributed to reactive tissue response to chronic irritation and trauma caused by a poorly fitted partial or complete prosthesis [13]. Prevalence of epulis fissuratum lesions was found to be 4.3% in Chilean population [22].

Treatment: Surgical excision and construction of a new denture adequate for the newly established mucosal contours. Excision can be performed by either conventional surgical approaches or by use of laser.

2.4 Inflammatory papillary hyperplasia

Localization: Inflammatory papillary hyperplasia of the palate is a benign epithelial proliferation that develops in patients who have complete acrylic maxillary dentures. Lesions are mostly seen in the hard palate. In few examples, they could be detected also in the lower jaw.

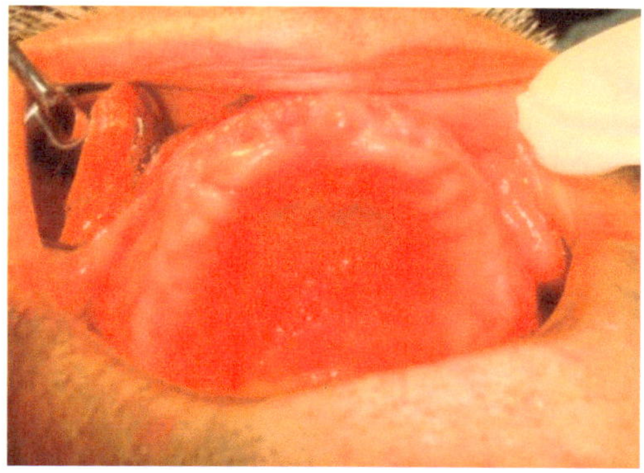

Figure 5.
Inflammatory papillary hyperplasia on the hard palate.

Clinical features: Inflammatory papillary hyperplasia lesions are generally asymptomatic and have color spectrums varying from red to pink. It presents as hyperplastic nodules 3–4mm wide, with erythematous and cobblestone appearance (**Figure 5**).

Etiology: Most often, patients wearing removable upper dentures show symptoms of inflammatory papillary hyperplasia. But rarely, it can be seen also in maxillary normal dentition. Pathogenic etiology is unclear. Continuous usage of prosthesis without night rest, inadequate denture flange edges, poor oral hygiene habits, allergic reactions against denture liners, abuse of tobacco, senility, and several systemic reactions are other reasons [6].

These dentures are often old, ill-fitting, badly cleaned, and worn all the time.

Treatment: Surgical excision and construction of a new denture. Different techniques have been described, including supra-periosteal excision, the bladeloop technique, or electrosurgery, with or without soft tissue grafts, cryosurgery, and laser [8]. Iegami et al. [23], reported that inflammatory papillary hyperplasia could completely be eliminated by the generated pressure combined with antioxidant and anti-inflammatory pastes and following this, a new set of complete dentures could be delivered to the patient.

2.5 Denture stomatitis

Localization: Denture stomatitis is seen under ill-fitting total or partial dentures.

Clinical features: It is characterized by diffuse erythema, edema, and sometimes petechiae and white spots that represent accumulations or Candida hyphae (**Figure 6**). Denture stomatitis is usually asymptomatic.

Etiology: Mechanical irritation from *C. albicans* dentures or a tissue response to microorganisms living beneath the dentures.

Treatment: Improvement of denture fit, oral hygiene, and topical or systemic antifungals or tissue disinfection by diode laser irradiation [3]. In the management of denture stomatitis, a more conservative approach regarding the usage of mouth rinses was advised by Koray et al. [19], in order to prevent the adverse effects and complications of systemic drugs.

2.6 Traumatic ulcers

Localization: Presence of traumatic ulcers is a relatively common finding in dental practice. Such lesions arise from trauma related to bite of buccal mucosa, lateral border of the tongue or lips during chewing. Traumatic ulcers seen in the mucobuccal folds

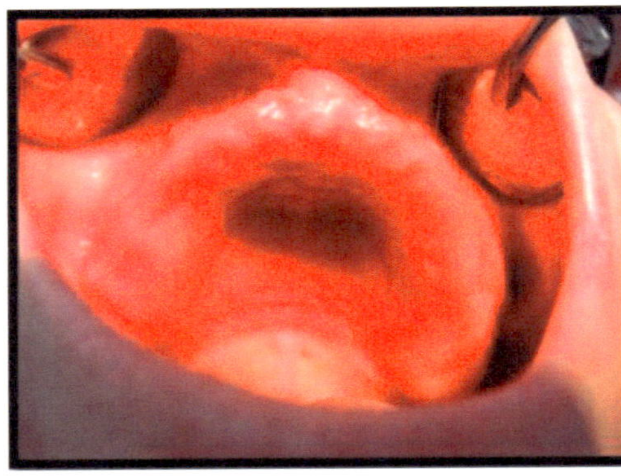

Figure 6.
Denture stomatitis located on the denture-bearing area of maxilla.

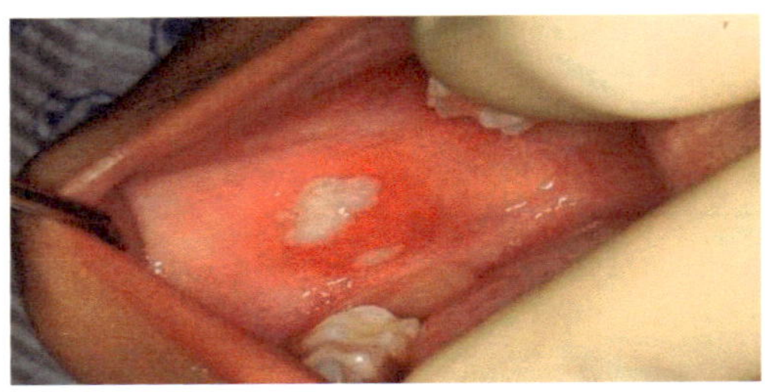

Figure 7.
Traumatic ulcer after accidental mucosal biting.

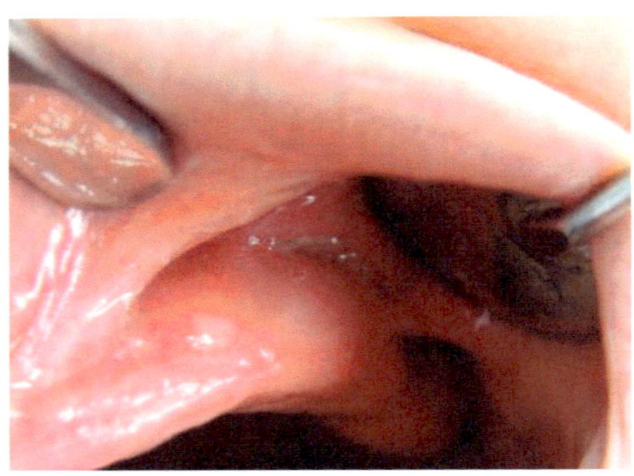

Figure 8.
Traumatic ulcer caused by sharp edges of prosthesis.

and gingiva are related to different irritant factors such as hard foods and inappropriate hard brushing. Traumatic ulcer due to lip biting after inferior dental nerve block is seen on the lower lip. During orthodontic treatment, traumatic ulcers can occur especially on the buccal mucosa due to the irritation of braces or appliance wires.

Clinical features: Traumatic ulcers could be of solitary shallow or deep discontinuity type showing on the epithelium and are associated with peripheral keratosis of mild to severe degree [2]. The bottom of the ulcerative lesions is made of whitish or yellow pseudomembrane. Upon elimination of the causative factor, often the ulcer heals with or without scar depending on the extent of the damage occurred.

Etiology: They could originate from accidental mucosal biting (**Figure 7**), sharp edges of prosthesis (**Figure 8**), sharp or pointed food stuff (**Figure 9**), during

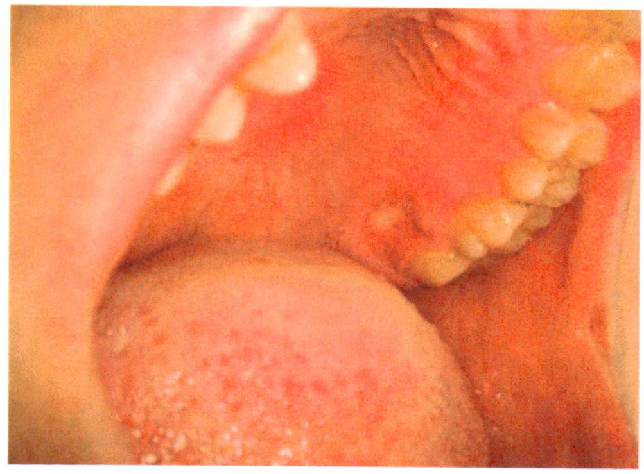

Figure 9.
Traumatic ulcer caused by sharp or puncturing food stuff.

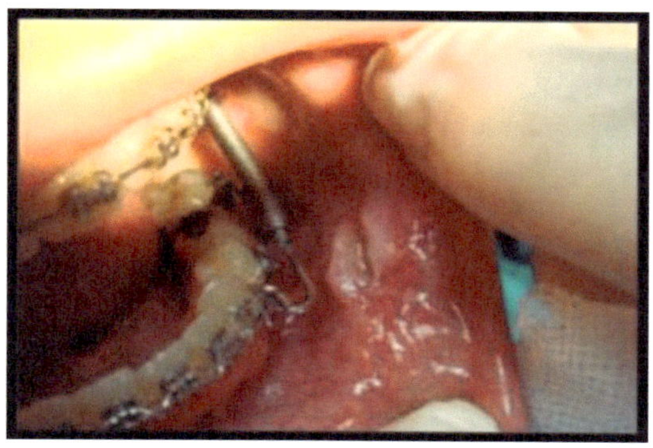

Figure 10.
Traumatic ulcers during orthodontic treatment.

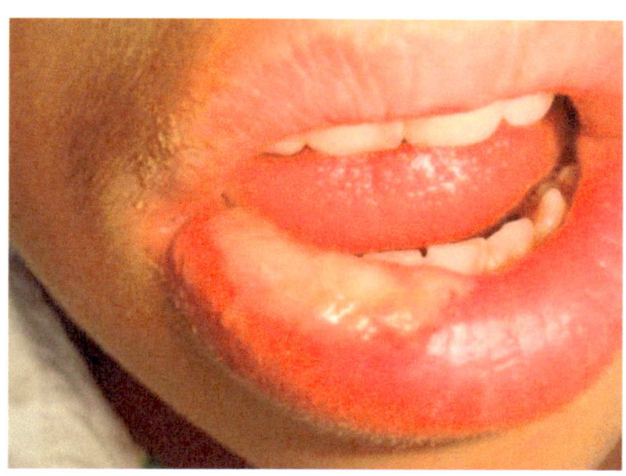

Figure 11.
Lip biting after injection of local anesthetic solutions.

orthodontic treatment (**Figure 10**), lip biting after injection of local anesthetic solutions (**Figure 11**), neonatal teeth (**Figure 12**), or faulty tooth brushing [1]. During dental treatments, iatrogenic damages can result in traumatic ulcer formation. Some medical treatments can cause oral ulcerations, such as brutal intubation for general anesthesia, ENT surgeries, or endoscopic interventions and iatrogenic malpractice applications. A high prevalence of traumatic ulcer of about 21.5% was reported among lower classes of Brazilian population [24]. Most prevalent types of lesions were reported to be traumatic ulcer and actinic cheilitis (7.5% for each) [25]. Among the

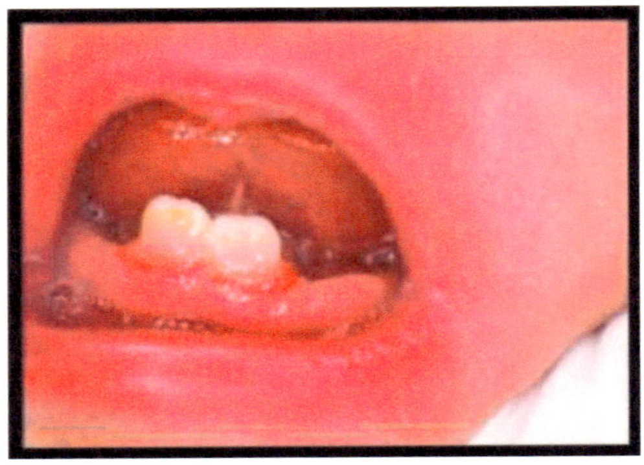

Figure 12.
Traumatic ulcer caused by neonatal teeth.

etiological factors of traumatic ulcers could be mentioned traumas caused by bites, dental appliances, inappropriate tooth brushing, misfit of removable partial or total dentures, irritating caries edges, malocclusion and puncturing restorations [25].

Treatment: Most often, traumatic ulcers can heal spontaneously and uneventfully without complications in a brief period of time. But, in case of persistent traumatic factors, such as presence of sharp tooth morphology, cutting edges of restorations, and puncturing appliance contours, especially inadequate surfaces of removable prosthesis, continuous trauma arising from above-mentioned causes can lead to formation of chronic ulcers.

2.7 Recurrent aphthous stomatitis

Localization: Non-keratinized oral mucosa is most frequently affected.

Clinical features: Recurrent lesions related to multifactorial chronic inflammation named as recurrent aphthous stomatitis (RAS) exhibit round or ovoid shape, pseudomembrane-covered ulcerations on the non-keratinized oral mucosa. Ulcers are surrounded by erythematous halo with superficial necrotic center and they are painful [10] (**Figure 13**).

Etiology: RAS is a complicated condition and the precise etiology still remains unknown. Several predisposing factors have been reported, such as trauma allergy, genetic predisposition, endocrine disturbances, emotional stress, and hematological deficiencies. Detailed examination of RAS history can explore the original etiology [27].

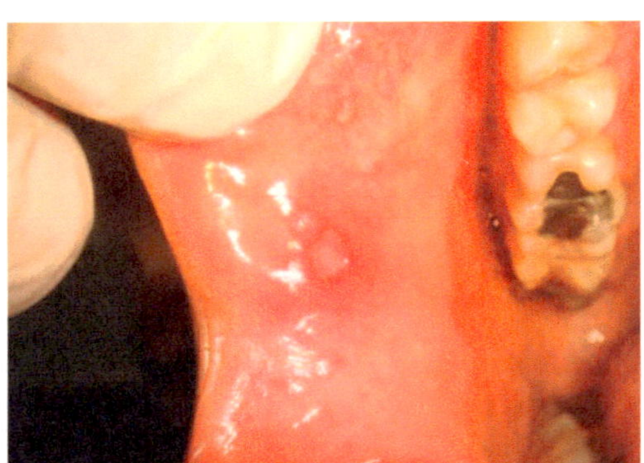

Figure 13.
Recurrent aphthous stomatitis on the buccal mucosa.

Treatment: The real etiological factors of RAS are still unclear and all treatment strategies are symptomatic. Fruit consumption would be useful to replace antioxidants via vitamin replenishment. Topical therapies such as mouth rinses are preferred as they have less risk of adverse effects [26, 27]. Pain relief is the main strategy of treatment. Anti-inflammatory coverage and reduction in function helps to decrease lesion duration, frequency, and recurrence. Topically applied medicaments such as antibiotics, local analgesics, glucocorticoids, astringents, hyaluronic acid gel, and low-level laser therapy are treatments of choice [10].

2.8 Nicotine stomatitis (smoker's palate)

Localization: Nicotine stomatitis is a common tobacco-related type of keratosis that exclusively occurs on the hard palate.

Clinical features: The palatal mucosa initially appears with redness. Subsequently, around the minor salivary gland ducts with inflamed and dilated orifices, many micronodules of punctate red centers form and make diffuse, grayish-white color wrinkles [5]. This type of lesion is not precancerous.

Etiology: Elevated temperature, rather than the tobacco chemicals, is responsible for this lesion. Among elderly Indian and Thailandian people, the general oral mucosal lesion type is smoker's palate with an incidence of 43%. Lesions mostly involve maxillary hard palate region with a prevalence of 23.1% [17, 18].

Treatment: Cessation of smoking.

2.9 Lip-licking dermatitis

Localization: Lips and its surrounding dermis

Clinical features: Erythematous lesions involve perioral skin and lips. Lesions may be associated with skin peeling, crusting, and fissuring to different degrees (**Figure 14**). Most often a burning sensation is present [11].

Etiology: Chronic licking

Treatment: Elimination of licking, and topical steroids.

2.10 Traumatic fibroma

Localization: The most common sites of traumatic fibroma are the tongue, buccal mucosa, and lower labial mucosa.

Traumatic or irritation fibroma is a common benign exophytic and reactive oral lesion that develops secondary to injury.

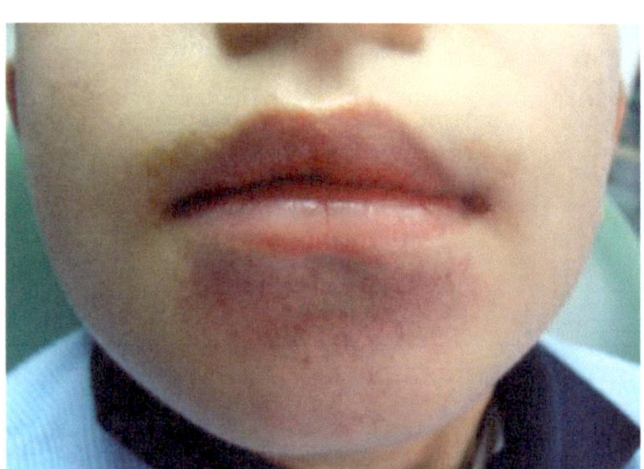

Figure 14.
Lip-licking dermatitis due to sucking a ball all day.

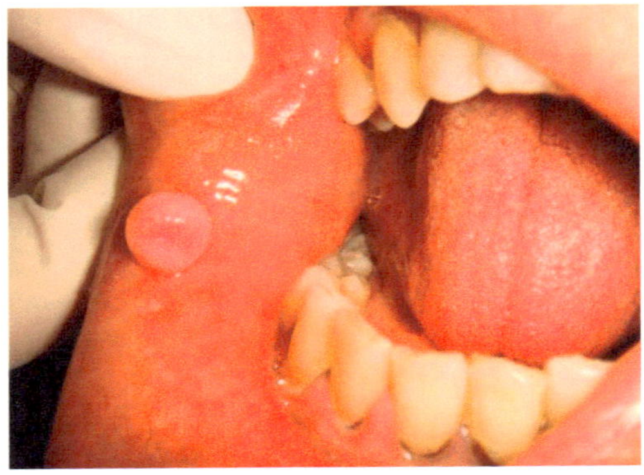

Figure 15.
Traumatic fibroma of the buccal mucosa.

Clinical features: Lesions are shown as broad-based, with light color in respect to neighboring normal tissue, superficially whitish as the secondary trauma causes formation of hyperkeratotic ulcerative surface.

Etiology: Recurrent repair process triggers the formation of fibromas which are accompanied by granulation and scar tissue. Fibroma is a result of a chronic repair process that includes granulation tissue and scar formation resulting in a fibrous submucosal mass. After surgical removal, recurrence may happen if repetitive trauma factor is not eliminated. Otherwise, lesions do not have malign neoplastic character and risk of repeated lesion formation [14] (**Figure 15**). According to Sangle et al. [28], traumatic fibroma with an incidence of 36.5% is the most common clinical lesion type; whereas histologically, the fibrous hyperplasia was found to be the most common one with a recurrence of 37.4%. Clinically, lesions with reactive characteristics may be sessile (51%) or pedunculated (49%) [28].

Treatment: Surgical excision.

2.11 Trauma associated with sexual practice

Localization: Oro-genital stimulation has become a popular practice during the last few decades and this is more common among homosexual males and females

Clinical features: This generally manifests as erythema, ecchymosis, or petechiae in the soft palate. These lesions may be noticed during routine oral examinations.

Etiology: Dentists should be aware of the reason and oral symptoms of lesions related to oro-genital sex habit. Among oro-genital sex actions, the most traumatic one is so called "fellatio" where male genital organ is taken into the mouth of partner to suck it and can cause lacerations to buccal mucosa and cheeks [2].

Treatment: The lesions are generally asymptomatic and heal within 7–10 days.

3. Chemical injuries of the oral mucosa

3.1 Chemical burn

Localization: Gingiva and mucobuccal folds are main localization regions of such lesions.

Clinical features: The wounds have irregular shape and white color, are overlaid by a pseudomembrane, and are very painful. Lesions can cover an extended area. If the lesions are contacted shortly, a shallow whitish and wrinkled appearance occurs. Brief contacts cannot cause necrosis [5].

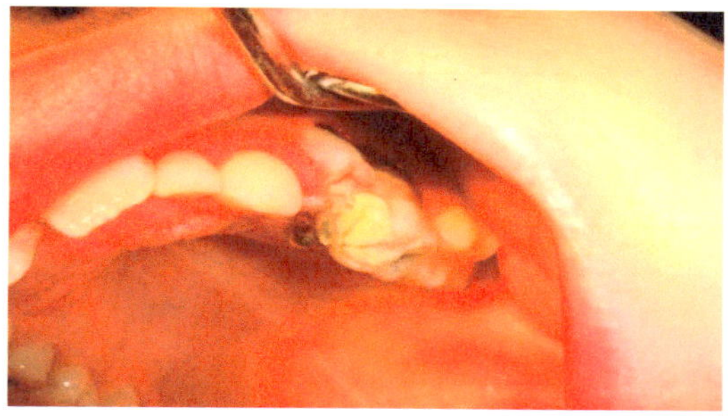

Figure 16.
Acid/arsenic injury.

Etiology: Caustic chemical and drug materials when they come in contact with the oral mucosa are often very irritating and cause direct mucosal trauma. Inappropriate usage of medications, such as aspirin application onto the neighboring mucosa of painful teeth with decay, may result in mucosal trauma. Iatrogenically, during dental treatments irrigant solutions (sodium hypochlorite or formalin) or some endodontic pastes with arsenic can irritate the mucosa [2] (**Figure 16**). However, such injuries are not very common since the introduction of rubber dam in dental practice.

Treatment: The best treatment of chemical burns of the oral cavity is prevention. The proper use of a rubber dam during endodontic procedures reduces the risk of iatrogenic chemical burns. Superficial burns of mucosa can heal in a short period of time (within 1 or 2 weeks) as the turn-over of oral mucosa is very high [5]. Oral surgery and antibiotics are necessary in very rare cases. Gel with hyaluronic acid can accelerate the healing process. Possible treatments after chemical injuries, in relation with the severity of wounds, are topical and intralesional corticosteroid applications, caustic acid ingestion, commissuroplasty, mucosal flaps, free radial forearm flap and free jejunal graft, surgeries made with electrocautery or soft tissue laser, and wound coverage by periodontal pack [29].

3.2 Post-anesthetic ulceration of palate

Localization: Post-anesthetic ulceration due to dental nerve block is seen on palatal mucosa. Ischemic necrosis of tissues may follow injections of local anesthetics. This can be due to the irritating nature of a solution, pressure from large volumes, or constriction of the vasculature by vasopressors [30, 31].

Clinical features: The floor of the ulcer is covered with grayish-white necrotic slough with sloping edge and erythematous margins; on palpation, the ulcer is slightly tender with no indurations present.

Etiology: Post-anesthetic ulceration can occur following the rapid injection of local anesthetic solutions, particularly those containing a vasoconstrictor.

Treatment: Management is usually conservative. It mainly consists of reassuring the patient, prescribing analgesics, and combination of topical antiseptic and anesthetic preparations. Healing generally occurs within 8–10 days after the onset of the lesion. Rarely surgical intervention is necessary when ulcer does not heal. An oral protective emollient orabase paste can also be prescribed [7].

3.3 Contact allergic stomatitis

Localization: Contact area of oral mucosa due to denture base materials, restorative materials, mouthwashes, dentifrices, chewing gums, food, and other substances. Various chemical or natural agents in contact with the mucosa can irritate and cause

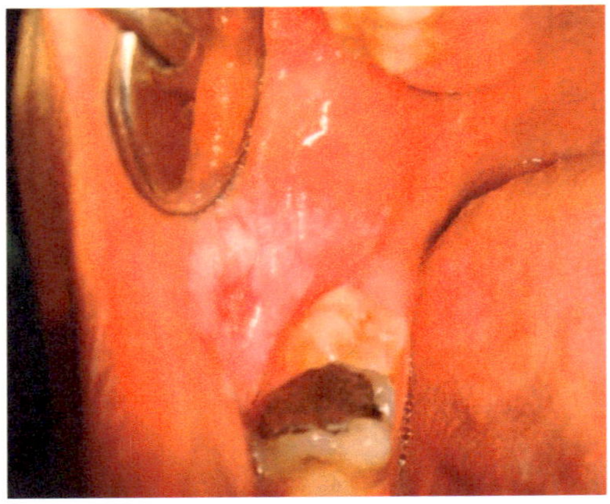

Figure 17.
Contact allergic stomatitis due to amalgam.

contact stomatitis. For example, cinnamaldehyde or cinnamon essential oil, which are commonly used as flavoring agents in foods, beverages, candies, and hygiene products by contact with mucosal surfaces, may trigger the formation of allergic stomatitis [32].

Clinical features: Diffuse erythema, edema, occasionally small vesicles, and shallow erosions appear immediately after contact with the allergen on the affected mucosal surfaces. Lesions are associated with burning symptom. In chronic allergies, whitish, hyperkeratotic, erythematous lesions form [11] .

Etiology: Denture base materials, restorative materials like amalgam (**Figure 17**), mouthwashes, dentifrices, chewing gums, food, and other substances may be responsible.

Treatment: Contact allergic stomatitis can be diagnosed by an accurate examination and clear understanding of medical history of the patient. Clinician's diagnostic ability and experience are highly important to avoid further unnecessary examinations, invasive and expensive diagnostic procedures [32]. Treatments include removal of suspected allergens, and use of topical or systemic corticosteroids, antihistamines.

4. Radiation injuries

4.1 Oral mucositis

Localization: Developments in oncology have led to improved survival rates for different cancers. Unfortunately, those treatment regimens have side effects such as formation of oral mucosal lesions. The most common wound type during chemotherapy is oral mucositis which appears by inflamed erosive or ulcerative lesions on mucosal surfaces in the oral cavity [33]. Generally, buccal mucosa is affected by radiation treatment of head and neck tumors [15].

Clinical features: After radiotherapy, at the end of first week, the first oral manifestations can appear. Lesions are erythematous and edematous. In the following days, ulcerative erosions with whitish-yellow exuadate appear. As salivary glands are involved, xerostomia occurs and is followed by tongue papillary changes with loss of taste, burning sensation, and pain during function. Speech is also affected negatively [11].

Etiology: Chemotherapy, radiotherapy, or their combinations can lead oral mucositis. The majority of patients (approximately 20–40%) receiving conventional chemotherapy regimens for solid tumors, in relation to the dose and cytotoxicity of the drug used, have oral mucositis. It is a side effect of radiation treatment of head and neck tumors.

Treatment: Supportive care, cessation of radiation treatment, B-complex vitamins, and sometimes low doses of corticosteroids are suggested.

4.2 Actinic chellitis

Localization: This type of lower lip lesion is mainly caused by solar irradiation (chronic or excessive exposure to sun light) [35]. Actinic cheilitis (AC) generally involves vermillion border of lower lip.

Clinical features: At the beginning, vermillion border of the lower lip is involved with mild erythema associated with edema, dryness, and fine desquamation. In later phases, smooth epithelium, small whitish-gray areas mixed with red regions, and scaly formations appear. Thin nodules and erosive surfaces may develop with time. The lesions could be precancerous [11].

Etiology: Long-term exposure to sunlight can lead to AC. People exposed to sun light exhibited AC with a prevalence of 9.16%. AC is more frequent among those patients who were exposed to solar irradiation more than 10 years, compared to those who were exposed for less than 10 years. AC is mostly seen in Caucasian males over 50 years of age.

Treatment: Surgical and non-surgical treatment options of AC are available. Surgical treatment or vermilionectomy is an invasive treatment choice and may include some side effects, such as secondary wound healing with delayed re-epithelialization, non-aesthetic appearance of lip, pain during the healing phase, edema, secondary infection, scarring, and disaesthesia [37]. Conventional surgical intervention or electrosurgery, laser ablation, and cryosurgery are alternative methods [38]. Except scalpel vermilionectomy, the other surgical methods mainly do not permit the histopathological examination of all tissues removed as they change the protein nature of specimen by thermal side effects [36, 38]. Among non-surgical therapies include the usage of topical pharmacotherapy with 5-fluorouracil, trichloroacetic acid, imiquimod, ingenol mebutate, and diclofenac. The non-surgical approach is less invasive and has fewer secondary effects. But contrarily, in a systematic review by Carvalho et al. [34], the surgical treatment was found to be more favorable than non-surgical for AC. However, it is very important to protect lips from sunlight.

5. Electrical and thermal burn

5.1 Electrical burn

Localization: Commissures of the mouth often result in severe facial scarring and deformation. Most commissural electrical burns involve mucosa, submucosa, muscle, nerve, and vascular tissue.

Clinical features: Damage made accidentally to lingual or/and labial arteries can cause abundant bleeding. When burned tissues spontaneously start to loosen or slough and occasional trauma occurs, this type of bleeding happens. Generally, this is observed 3–4 days after burn injury [12]. Pressure should be applied to the hemorrhage site to stop the bleeding and the patient should be taken to the nearest hospital emergency room for definitive care.

Etiology: The majority of electrical burns are home accidents. Generally, children play with live electric extension cables/cords and may contact or suck them and are injured by current. Especially in the cable/plug junctions, in non-fitted appliance plugs, the electric current flows through tongue or oral cavity when they are in contact with saliva, and the electric energy burns oral tissues. Children under three years of age are mostly affected by this type of injury [12].

Treatment: Whatever is the severity of burned injury, the basic treatment strategy involves pain relief, infection control, and acceleration of wound repair [39]. Application of antibiotic ointments to the burn area has been recommended by some authors. Systemic antibiotics are recommended by most clinicians to prevent wound infection. Facial disfigurement takes place if splints are not applied. Microstomia reduces mouth opening, renders oral hygiene difficult, and decreases functions of speech and chewing. Most of the cases need plastic surgery. [12].

5.2. Thermal burn

Localization: Oral mucosa, especially tongue and palatal mucosa.

Clinical features: Clinically, the condition appears as a red or white, painful erythema that may undergo desquamation, leaving erosions (**Figure 18**). In excessive damage to tissues, necrosis could appear. In mild lesions, wounds can heal spontaneously within a week [11].

Etiology: Thermal burns mostly happen by accidental ingestion of hot substances. High incidence of thermal burns with a prevalence of 24.6% is seen among children and young patients [40]. Usually caused due to contact with very hot foods, liquids, hot metal objects or iatrogenic usage of lasers (diodes, Nd:YAG, Er:YAG or CO_2), piezoelectric surgery, or electrosurgery devices.

Treatment: No treatment is required for simple lesions. Care should be taken in deep lesions to avoid contamination during healing period. Saline would be prescribed to accelerate wound healing and avoid bacterial ingrowth. Ozone therapy and laser biomodulation could help for good prognosis. In severe damages, prophylactic antibiotic coverage is recommended. In hard tissue damages related to thermal burn, the necrotic area should be removed surgically in order to avoid damage to surrounding vital tissues and obtain blood supply for repair and subsequent regeneration.

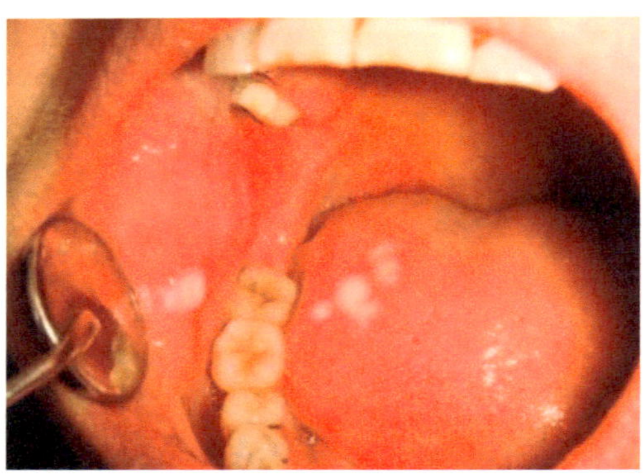

Figure 18.
Thermal iatrogenic burn during aerator usage.

Author details

Meltem Koray[1]* and Tosun Tosun[2]

1 Department of Oral and Maxillofacial Surgery, Dental School, Istanbul University, Istanbul, Turkey

2 Department of Oral and Maxillofacial Surgery, Dental School, Istanbul Aydin University, Istanbul, Turkey

*Address all correspondence to: mkoray@istanbul.edu.tr

References

[1] Ahmed A, Zardawi FM, Mohammed GN. Oral mucosal and periodontal changes of patients under treatment with manual invisalign and fixed labial orthodontic appliances. IOSR Journal of Dental and Medical Sciences. 2015;**14**(3):102-107

[2] Ariyawardana A. Traumatic oral mucosal lesions: A mini review and clinical update. Oral Health and Dental Management. 2014;**13**(2):254-259

[3] deSennaa AM, Vieirab MMF, Machado-de-Senac RM, Bertolind AO, Núñeze SC, Ribeirof MS. Photodynamic inactivation of *Candida* ssp. on denture stomatitis. A clinical trial involving palatal mucosa and prosthesis disinfection. Photodiagnosis and Photodynamic Therapy. 2018;**22**:212-216

[4] El Toum S, Cassia A, Bouchi N, Kassab I. Prevalence and distribution of oral mucosal lesions by sex and age categories: A retrospective study of patients attending Lebanese school of dentistry. International Journal of Dentistry. 2018:6. DOI: 10.1155/2018/4030134

[5] Greenberg MS, Glick M. Oral Medicine Diagnosis & Treatment Burket's Tenth Edition. BC Decker Inc.; 2003

[6] Gual-Vaqués P, Jané-Salas E, Egido-Moreno S, Ayuso-Montero R, MaríRoig A, López-López J. Inflammatory papillary hyperplasia: A systematic review. Medicina Oral, Patología Oral y Cirugía Bucal. 2017;**22**(1):e36-e42

[7] Gupta R, Garg M, Pawah S, Gupta A. Postanesthetic ulceration of palate: A rare complication. National Journal of Maxillofacial Surgery. 2016;**7**(1):86-88

[8] Infante-Cossio P, Martinez-de-Fuentes R, Torres-Carranza E, Gutierrez-Perez JL. Inflammatory papillary hyperplasia of the palate: Treatment with carbon dioxide laser, followed by restoration with an implant-supported prosthesis. British Journal of Oral and Maxillofacial Surgery. 2007;**45**:658-660

[9] Kashani HG, Mackenzie IC, Kerber PE. Cytology of *Linea alba* using a filter imprint technique. Clinical Preventive Dentistry. 1980;**2**:21-24

[10] Koray M, Ofloglu D, Senemtasi A, İşsever H, Yaltirik M. The efficacy of hyaluronic acid gel in pain control of recurrent aphthous stomatitis. International Journal of Dentistry and Oral Science. 2016;**3**(6):273-275

[11] Laskaris G. Pocket Atlas of Oral Dseases. New York: Thieme Med. Publ; 1998

[12] LeCompteand EJ, Goldman BM. Oral lectrical burns in children-early treatment and appliance fabrication. Pediatric Dentistry. 1982;**4**(4):333-337

[13] Mohan RPS, Verma S, Singh U, Agarwal N. Epulis fissuratum: Consequence of ill-fitting prosthesis. BML Case Reports. 2013. DOI: 10.1136/bcr-2013-200054

[14] Rathva VJ. Traumatic fibroma of tongue. BMJ Case Reports. 2013. DOI: 10.1136/bcr-2012-008220

[15] Sonis ST, Costa JW Jr. Oral complications of radiotherapy. In: Kufe DW, Pollock RE, Weichselbaum RR, et al., editors. Holland-Frei Cancer Medicine. 6th ed. Hamilton (ON): BC Decker; 2003

[16] Tortorici S, Corrao S, Natoli G, Difalco P. Prevalence and distribution of oral mucosal non-malignant lesions in the western Sicilian population. Minerva Stomatologica. 2016;**65**(4):191-206

[17] Intapa C, Na Ayudhya CC, Puangsombat A, Boonmoon B, Janyasurin T, Tonum U. Prevalence of oral mucosal lesions in geriatric patients living in lower Northern Thailand: A 10 years retrospective study. Journal of International Dental and Medical Research. 2017;**10**(3):868-871

[18] Patil S, Doni B, Maheshwari S. Prevalence and distribution of oral mucosal lesions in a geriatric Indian population. Canadian Geriatrics Journal. 2015;**18**(1):11-14

[19] Koray M, Ak G, Kürklü E, İşsever H, Tanyeri G, Kulekçi G, et al. Fluconazole and/or hexetidine for management of oral candidiasis associated with denture-induced stomatitis. Oral Disease. 2005;**11**:309-313

[20] Woo SB, Lin D. Morsicatio mucosae oris—A chronic oral frictional keratosis, not a leukoplakia. Journal of Oral and Maxillofacial Surgery. 2009;**67**:140-142

[21] Neville BW, Damm DD, Allen CM, Bouquot JE. Oral and Maxillofacial Pathology. Philadelphia: Saunders; 2009

[22] Rivera C, Droguett D, Arenas-Márquez MJ. Oral mucosal lesions in a chilean elderly population: A retrospective study with a systematic review from thirteen countries. Journal of Clinical and Experimental Dentistry. 2017;**9**(2):e276-83

[23] Iegami CM, Tamaki R, Neto PT. A 5-week non-surgical approach towards denture induced hyperplasia. The Open Dentistry Journal. 2017;**11**:151-154

[24] Vieira-Andrade RG, Zuquim Guimarães Fde F, Vieira Cda S, Freire ST, Ramos-Jorge ML, Fernandes AM. Oral mucosa alterations ina socioeconomically deprived region: Prevalence and associated factors. Brazilian Oral Research. 2011;**25**(5):393-400

[25] Cury PR, Araujo NS, Oliveira MGA, Santos JN. Association between oral mucosal lesions and crack and cocaine addiction in men: A cross-sectional study. Environmental Science and Pollution Research. 2018;**25**:19801-19807

[26] Altenburg A, El-Haj N, Micheli C, et al. The treatment of chronic recurrent oral aphthous ulcers. Deutsches Ärzteblatt International. 2014;**111**:665-673

[27] Saikaly SK, Saikaly TS, Saikaly LE. Recurrent aphthous ulceration: A review of potential causes and novel treatments. Journal of Dermatological Treatment. 2018. DOI: 10.1080/09546634.2017.1422079

[28] Sangle VA, Pooja VK, Holani A, Shah N, Chaudhary M, Khanapure S. Reactive hyperplastic lesions of the oral cavity: A retrospective survey study and literature review. Indian Journal of Dental Research. 2018;**29**(1):61-66

[29] Rallan M, Malhotra G, Rallan NS, et al. BML Case Reports Published online. DOI: 10.1136/bcr-2013- 009083

[30] Malamed SF. Handbook of Local Anesthesia. 5th ed. St. Louis: The C.V. Mosby Co; 2004

[31] Becker DE, Reed KL. Local anesthetics: Review of pharmacological considerations. Anesthesia Progress. 2012;**59**:90-101

[32] Vivas APM, Migliari DA. Cinnamon-induced oral mucosal contact reaction. The Open Dentistry Journal. 2015;**9**:257-259

[33] Lalla RV, Saunders DP, Peterson DE. Chemotherapy or radiation-induced oral mucositis. Dental Clinics of North America. 2014;**58**:341-349

[34] Carvalho MV, Moraes SLD, Lemos CAA, Santiago JJF, Vasconcelos BC,

Pellizzer EP. Surgical versus non-surgical treatment of actinic cheilitis: A systematic review and meta-analysis. Oral Diseases. 2018. DOI: 10.1111/odi.12916

[35] Gomes JO, de Vasconcelos Carvalho M, Fonseca FP, Gondak RO, Lopes MA, Vargas PA. CD1a+ and CD83+ Langerhans cells are reduced in lower lip squamous cell carcinoma. Journal of Oral Pathology & Medicine. 2016;**45**(6):433-439. DOI: 10.1111/jop.12389

[36] Calcaianu N, Popescu SA, Diveica D, Lascar I. Surgical attitude in premalignant lesions and malignant tumors of the lower lip. Journal of Medicine and Life. 2015;**8**(1):109-111

[37] Castiñeiras I, Del Pozo J, Mazaira M, Rodríguez-Lojo R, Fonseca E. Actinic cheilitis: Evolution to squamous cell carcinoma after carbon dioxide laser vaporization. A study of 43 cases. Journal of Dermatological Treatment. 2010;**21**(1):49-53. DOI: 10.3109/09546630902887203

[38] Vieira RA, Minicucci EM, Marques ME, Marques SA. Actinic cheilitis and squamous cell carcinoma of the lip: Clinical, histopathological and immunogenetic aspects. Anais Brasileiros de Dermatologia. 2012;**87**(1):105-114

[39] Kang S, Kufta K, Sollecito TP, Panchal N. A treatment algorithm for the management of intraoral burns: A narrative review. Burns. 2018;**44**:1065-1076

[40] Cowan D, Ho B, Sykes KJ, Wei JL. Pediatric oral burns: A ten-year review of patient characteristics, etiologies and treatment outcomes. International Journal of Pediatric Otorhinolaryngology. 2013;**77**(8):1325-1328